IN THE MOMENT

A Practical Guide
to Movement and
Improvisation
for Actors

SARAH HICKLER

Published by The Joy Press
New York, NY

ISBN 978-0-9727450-4-8

Cover and interior design and typesetting by Jane Tenenbaum
Front cover photo by Bob Raymond

—

Printed in the United States of America

ACKNOWLEDGMENTS

I would like to express my deep gratitude to Merry Conway, whose editorial assistance, guidance and support made this book possible. Her work and insightful inquiry have informed and enriched my life and work beyond words. I am also indebted to Susan Dibble who first introduced me to movement for actors, and encouraged me to teach. Her artistry in classrooms and on stage continually inspires me.

While the others who have influenced my work are too numerous to mention, I am forever indebted to Ruth Zaporah for teaching and guiding me over the past two decades through the endless terrain of Action Theater™, Janet Adler and Zoe Avstreih for guiding me in the practice of Authentic Movement, and my colleagues at Shakespeare & Company.

I would like to extend a heartfelt thank you to Cassandra Tunick and Debra Bluth for additional editorial assistance; and to Louis Colaianni, Owen Walker, Michele LeBrun, Lisa Hickler, and my colleagues and students at Emerson College.

Dear Hannah —
Congratulations —
on a wonderful 4 years here,
for the beginning of your career,
and for being an overall
wonderful human being!
Much love & respect,
Ted Hewlett

CONTENTS

INTRODUCTION

I taught myself how to sail on a pond in Maine where I have spent my summers since I was born. Through trial and error I learned that thinking and effort alone would not keep the small sailboat from capsizing in strong winds. I discovered that if I relaxed and breathed I could focus my attention on the cues of the wind and water, the feel of the sheet in my hand and the boat underneath me. That information coming to me through my senses invited immediate physical response. I experienced a sense of flight and grace as I sailed.

On other summer days I would ride a neighbor's unpredictable horse. The horse could read the subtlest shifts in my energy and attention. His response to my willful determination to gain control over him was to throw me off his back. I eventually figured out the collaborative nature of riding; if I relaxed my body and mind I could reciprocate the horse's full-bodied listening, and experience the power and beauty of this animal as we rode.

Both of these experiences filled me with awe — a combination of respect, wonder and a little fear. Being in direct relationship with these two forces of nature on those summer days helped me come into a more direct relationship with myself. I came to know the innate wisdom of the body and how to trust it as my guide. I also began to learn about the nature of collaboration and what it means to be present.

The same curiosity and passion that drew me to animal and element have drawn me into dance studios, theaters and classroom for over thirty years. I continue to apply those early lessons to my work in movement, physical improvisation, acting and directing. I experience the living impulse as a dynamic process of exchange — of collaboration, exploration, discovery and invention. This is true whether I am performing in front of an audience, rehearsing with a theater company, creating new work, or guiding actors in a studio.

Theater is a living, human exchange, immediate and in the present. Live people perform to a live audience. We call the work we do on stage a play, because it is play. Actor and audience collectively lend themselves to an imaginary world. At its best, theater engages all of our senses and sensibilities in a genuine experience of exchange that enlivens and illuminates both performer and audience.

Acting requires an ability to bring all of one's preparation, energy, and intention to bear in performance. In order to believably inhabit imaginary situations as actors do, they must be able to genuinely respond to internal and external stimulation visibly, viscerally, and in the moment. The challenge is to remain fully embodied and engaged, open and available in and to the present moment of experience. This takes training, practice, and skill. It is this availability and quality of attention in an actor that draws an audience in, can engage and keep them riveted, and has the potential to inspire.

A dynamic and alive presence is something I've heard referred to as "It" and "something special." It is. But it is not necessarily a mysterious attribute or innate talent. It requires a unique set of skills that can be learned, and that are not typically directly addressed in actor training. This manual addresses those skills. It is a progression of fifty-six exercises that represent key aspects of my approach to movement and physical improvisation for actors. At the core of this approach is training the internal muscles of attention and awareness necessary to genuinely show up — body, mind and spirit, in the present moment. This may sound obvious or simple, but it is a lifetime practice that is challenging, infinitely rewarding, and an essential component of actor training and performance.

Actors are the instruments of their art. In order to personify a character and function within imaginary circumstances, an actor needs to first come into a clearer relationship with him/herself. The progression of exercises in this manual offers a framework and foundation in which actors are able to establish a deeper rapport with themselves, each other, and the world around them. This approach engenders a ground of awareness firmly rooted in a body, mind, and self, so there is a facility ready to learn, fully engage, and to take action.

An Embodied Perspective

We live in a culture that values conceptual processes, such as logic and thinking, over body-based processes, such as sensing and feeling. Media and new technology in which electronic communication and participation in computer social networks are the norm reinforce this perspective. In this landscape, the written and spoken word seems to be increasingly perceived as our sole means of communication. We can use these electronic tools to communicate our thoughts and report on our experiences, but the body is increasingly left behind. The internal muscle that enables us to remain open and responsive as we negotiate the ever-changing contours of the present moment, and to communicate *from* that experience in full-bodied and emotionally connected expression seems to be atrophying.

The body is often described colloquially as a mechanical form. It is not uncommon in our culture to perceive and relate to the body as separate from our essential sense of self. Because of the cultural emphases on the cognitive, most of our attention is on our thoughts. We may so over-identify with our thoughts that we confuse the act of *thinking* for the act of *directly experiencing*. Thinking does shape our experiences, and our experiences do shape our thoughts. Yet experiencing and communicating from our experience is a full-bodied proposition. It is with and through the body that we sense, feel, experience, and communicate.

The body has its own logic and wisdom. The dynamic connection of mind and body is the source of our power, desires, passions, emotions, instincts, intuition, imagination, and creative impulses. Happily for those of us who specialize in body-based practices, exciting new findings in the field of neuroscience strongly reaffirm the mind/body connection.

The theater makes an enormous contribution to our understanding of what it means to be human. Actors, therefore, must be trained to inhabit a strong sense of the mind/body connection. In order to develop the physical, emotional, and mental agility necessary in their work, the actor needs to develop skills to reorient attention and expand awareness to the body. This enables us to access the depth and breadth of our inner resources, perceptual processes, and expressive potential. Actors' physical awareness and skills become more refined in the process outlined in this manual, but the primary focus is on developing a strong, flexible connection between the senses, feelings, imagination, and action. Through this process the mind becomes more tuned and oriented to the whole of experience.

In This Manual

Movement for actors is a broad field. Movement training needs to provide an understanding of many facets of physical work, and prepare actors for the variety of work they will encounter on stage. Like most who specialize in this area of training, I draw on a variety of methods and approaches, and cover a broad range of skills in my work — from basic physical awareness and conditioning, to character work and period styles, mask, and social dance. A number of excellent books and articles on movement for actors have been published in recent years that have significantly contributed to the understanding and practices in this important field. Yet no book can replace the experiential learning process necessary to practice and teach movement for actors.

This manual provides a starting place, and is a practical guide for teachers, professionals, and students of acting. It outlines key aspects of my approach to movement and physical improvisation, but does not represent all of my methods. The progression in this manual is intended to supplement, enrich, and inform movement curricula and the actor's process.

I have been teaching actors and theater educators for over twenty-five years, primarily in universities, professional theaters, and acting studios. My approach is geared towards those environments and populations. These exercises can be re-sequenced, or combined with other methods, or reframed for different contexts, ages, and levels of expertise.

This aspect of my approach to movement and physical improvisation does not represent a technique. There are no outside models of perfection to aspire to or imitate. These exercises encourage students to begin a dialogue with the body — to notice, listen, experience, and respond. Structures with specific guidelines are offered, and function much like the banks of a river. How the water flows within those banks is as unique as each individual.

The creative process is a state of ongoing somatic (body/mind) exploration, in which we — as sensing, feeling, thinking beings — investigate, experiment, and make discoveries. For many students of acting, especially those who have adopted a passive or consumer attitude to learning, this approach is new and helps prepare the ground for all of their actor training and work on stage.

The tendency to approach movement mechanically and to focus on producing results is common. In contrast, the methods in this manual redirect attention less on *what* one is doing, and more on *how* one is doing it. The quality of attention, intention, and impulse behind an action is key. Actors become more firmly rooted in a process of noticing, experiencing, and responding to and from their genuine experience. This results in strong, specific actions that are congruent with the actors' inner experiences.

Acting students eventually learn to trust that there is no one correct result in this approach to training. They potentially gain an inner muscle and appetite for the discomfort that often accompanies not knowing "the answers," and an appreciation for the nuances and contradictions that are part of an actor's training and process. They learn what it means to apply oneself to a process and practice instead of mechanically producing results. Through this they gain confidence in themselves and the legitimacy of their inner resources and experiences in their work. This is key to developing into intelligent, generous, and generative artists who can collaborate and fully participate in a creative process and in performance.

Part One addresses the actor coming into relationship with him/herself. It begins with centering and alignment and a series of exercises that reinforce moving from center. Tuning into the mechanics of the body, the senses, activating and engaging the imagination are emphasized, aiding clarity and specificity of actions and expressiveness of an experience.

In Part Two, an inner-directed movement process is introduced in which actors are guided to listen, respond, and give form to their internal landscape and impulses. In most of the sequences of exercises, the actor begins with the self, and then immediately extends awareness to include the environment and working in relationship to others.

Part Three introduces improvisational scores that emphasize partnering and ensemble work. In Parts Four and Five, I draw on my work in Action Theater™, a physical approach to improvisation that was developed by Ruth Zaporah. Action Theater is a system of training that combines and strengthens the connection between the body, voice, and language. Fundamental to this method is an embodied presence in performance, where the experience of the body informs the content of the moment, from moment to moment.[1] The focus is on developing a more fully physicalized relationship between the speaking body and the spoken word.

Many of the concepts central to my training in modern dance, yoga, Action Theater, Authentic Movement, Contact Improvisation, somatic body practices, movement forms that employ imagery such as Bhuto, Linklater Voice, and the training methods developed at Shakespeare and Company come through in these pages, as do the concepts, practices and words of my teachers.

---

[1] www.actiontheater.com

IN THE MOMENT

PART ONE

The Centered Body

Don't go outside your house to see flowers…
Inside your body there are flowers.
One flower has a thousand petals.
That will do for a place to sit.

— Kabir

Sequence 1: Preparing the Ground

We begin with sequences of exercises that introduce centering and alignment. Consciously centering and aligning is a physical, emotional, and mental practice of awareness. Dropping into center means dropping into the core of one's being. It is the source of our power, emotion, imagination, motivation, and creativity. It is the ground through which we take in and respond to our internal and external worlds, and a necessary component of what we call *presence*, on and off the stage. Living and working from a centered state can have a profound effect on our perception, experience, and sense of self.

Our physical awareness tends to be restricted to the surface of the front of the upper body and the face. When speaking, it is common to have excess energy and tension in the face, head, and neck. On stage this results in leaning forward, pushing the face forward, and shortening the back of the neck. This interferes with vocal production, breath, and accessing our full emotional range.

The physical center of gravity in the body is about two inches below the navel. When we extend our awareness into the core of the body and lower our center of gravity, the result is the release of excess tension and a deepening of the breath. This inspires greater emotional, mental, and physical flexibility, stability and balance. Centering is a unifying and grounding process that allows us to move as an integrated whole and experience a flow of energy. It engenders a sense of inner calm and stillness while actively engaged in activity.

An energetic awareness and connection to center is reinforced through the instructor's use of language and imagery, even in the most basic movement exercises. Repetition and constant reminders are necessary. Students quickly recognize this is an ongoing *practice* that extends outside studio exercises, and has implications that extend into all areas of their lives.

WAKING UP THE CORE

This is a simple centering exercise with which I begin and end almost every movement class. My students uniformly report appreciation for the ritual of doing this set sequence of movements. Coordinating the breath with movement is central to all of the exercises in this manual. Breath is the entrance to the body. When we breathe in we are taking in the world around us, and when we breathe out we are releasing energy into the world.

We do *Waking Up the Core* a few times as I guide students through the movement and breathing (Part I). Actors focus on the mechanics of the movements — how to initiate these simple movements, notice and release excess tension, and how to coordinate the actions with the breath. We then repeat the sequence with specific intentions and images (Part II). This affects the quality of the movement and experience of the mover. It is a starting place to connecting external action to internal states, and moving from center with clear intention and an active imagination.

Part I

1   Allow your breath to drop into your center and release out. Imagine energy radiating from your center up through your core and spine, and down your arms. As you breathe in, radiate your arms out to your side and up above your head. Bring your palms together over your head, fingers pointing straight up. Feel a little weight in your tailbone and see if you can sense if you are pushing your lower ribs forward or shortening your back. If so, release your rib cage and just let it float over your pelvis. Feel your feet on the floor. Hold this position as you release your breath.

2   Bending your elbows, bring your palms down in front of your heart-center (the center of your chest) as you breath in. Press your palms together, with your elbows out and in line with your hands and shoulders. Relax your shoulders, and gently press them down.

3 Extend your arms out in front of you, chest height, palms up, as you breathe out. Hold this position and breath in.

4 Open your arms out to the sides, keeping them at shoulder height, palms facing up, as you breathe out.

5 Raise your arms up slightly, palms up, as you breath in. Now turn your palms down towards the floor, elbows facing up, as you press your arms down to your side and breathe out.

Part II

1 Radiate your arms from your center, out and above your head, with your palms up, as if you were scooping energy up from the earth. You can bend your arms as you do this. Press your palms together over your head, arms straight, and sense how your hands are in a direct line above the crown of your head, fingers pointing up towards the heavens. There is strength in you and in this position. Gently press your feet into the floor.

2 Bring all that energy from the heavens down into your heart. Breathe into your heart center, and see if you can feel an expansion there.

3 Bring your energy out into the world from your heart. Your palms are up and open.

4 Generously extend your energy out into the world. As you open you arms to the side, imagine you are radiating energy and light from your heart, down your arms, and out your fingertips.

5 Now bring all this energy back to your center and the earth.

The tendency to approach movement exercises mechanically is common. Part II can help connect energy and intention with actions. There is a qualitative difference between mechanically opening your arms to the side, and radiating energy from your heart out your fingertips as you release the breath from the core of the body.

ISOLATIONS

Isolations encourage physical articulation. This warm up builds awareness of specific areas of the body referred to in the next exercise, *Standing Alignment*.

1 From the crown of your head, tilt your head to one side, bringing your ear directly towards your shoulder. Make sure your face is not turned up, down or back.

2 Keep your shoulders, ribs and chest still. Sensing the weight of your head, release your neck to allow your head to roll forward — chin down to chest. Release your breath as you do this.

3 From your crown, roll your head to the other side — ear towards the shoulder. Breathe in as you do this. Very gently press your entire shoulder girdle (collar bone, shoulder blades) down.

4 Feeling the weight of your head, continue to roll it: ear to one shoulder, head rolls forward, chin to chest, to the other side, ear to shoulder.

5 Place one hand on the center of your chest. Initiating from the center of your chest (between your sternum and your spine) gently press your chest forward, then back, then left and right. Let your shoulders just go along for the ride, and go slowly. See if you can keep your neck released, hips and tail bone still. Repeat a few times.

6 Now circle your upper body, initiating from your chest — forward to side to back to other side. Breathe.

7 Trace your rib cage with your finger from the front to the back. Trace your ribs up your front, right up to your collarbone. Place your hands around your sides on your lower ribs.

8 Move your whole rib cage to the right. Your spine, shoulders and head are just going along for the ride. Now move your rib cage to the left. Gently press your rib cage forward. As you do this, have a sense of a little weight in your tailbone. Now press your ribs back.

9 Breathe, and slowly circle your rib cage — front, side, back, side. See how slowly, smoothly and luxuriously you can do this.

10 Bend your knees slightly. Place your hands on your hips.

11 Release your jaw and breath through your mouth.

12 Keeping a sense of a little weight in your tailbone, slowly move your hips from left to right. Imagine you have wonderfully ample hips, or that you are wearing a big grass skirt like a Hula dancer. Breathe.

13 Now move your hips forward and back. Imagine the *bowl of your pelvis*[2] as you do this, as if you were spilling the contents of that bowl as it tips forward and back.

14 Now slowly circle your hips as if you were stirring something thick with your tailbone. Continue to relax your jaw and breathe through your mouth. See if you can allow energy out your eyes — a little twinkle or a hint of mischief — as if you were stirring up a bit of trouble with your tailbone.

STANDING ALIGNMENT

When first introducing actors to *Standing Alignment*, I bring in a model of a human skeleton to review with them. Investigating the model of the skeleton and then immediately investigating through touch and movement specific areas on our own and each other's bodies, such as the spine, pelvis, joints, the position of the skull in relationship to the spine, is very useful. Most acting students I have worked with have a limited knowledge of their anatomy. This process helps them visualize and sense their own skeletal system.

Standing Alignment is a relaxed and energized state in which you cultivate a sense of arrival and openness. When first doing this exercise you begin by waking up and messaging your own feet. The

---

2 When reviewing the skeleton with students, we look at the pelvic area — the sacrum, illium, pectineal line to the pubic bone — which forms a bowl-like shape.

tripod of the foot on which we stand is a triangle between the heels, outside of the feet and across the balls of the feet. Centering over the tripods of the feet, and awareness of weight pouring into the floor through the feet while standing allows you to release excess tension throughout your body, and to begin to let go of any sense of holding yourself up with the chest, neck and head, which is quite common.

1. Standing with feet parallel, align your feet under you hip sockets. You may want to put your hands on your hip bones and look down at your feet to see if they are actually parallel and aligned under your hip sockets. Close your eyes, and notice your breath dropping in and releasing out of the body. See if you can feel the gentle expansion and release in your belly, rib cage, chest, and spine as you breathe.

2. *Feet:* Bring your attention to your feet. Imagine the surfaces of the soles of your feet softening, and the bones of your feet spreading. Notice the surfaces of your feet that are in contact with the floor. See if you can sense if your weight is evenly distributed between your left and right foot. See if your weight is evenly distributed on the *tripod of your feet.* Experiment with making micro-adjustments from your center, moving your center slightly forward if you sense more weight in your heel, or slightly back if you sense more weight in the balls of your feet. Keep breathing.

3. *Legs:* Imagine a small pocket of air in your ankles. With your mind's eye trace the bones from your ankles to your knees. Soften your kneecaps and the backs of your knees. Your legs are straight, but the knees are not locked. (If necessary, I have students lock their knees and pull their kneecaps up for a moment so they can more easily sense the release in the knee). Trace the bones from your knees into your hip sockets. See if you can release your inner thighs, and sense a softening in your hip sockets. Feel how the bones of your legs are balanced on the tripod of your feet. Allow the muscles of your legs to relax, and let your strong bones support you. Check in with your feet and see if they are relaxed.

4. *Pelvis:* Now imagine the bowl of your pelvis floating on top of your legs. Bring your breath to your belly, and allow the belly to relax. Imagine a small weight on your tailbone, and allow your

lower back to widen and release. Imagine your breath dropping into your belly about two inches bellow your navel.

5   *Ribs:* Feel your rib cage expand and release on every breath. Your ribs begin under your collarbone, and extend down toward your waist. They curve around your sides to your back and are connected to your spine, and to your sternum in the front of your body. Imagine you can rinse the inside of your rib cage with your breath — back, sides and front. Sense how the rib cage is floating over your pelvis. See if you can sense your lowest rib in your back and imagine you are massaging it with your breath.

6   *Upper chest:* Bring your attention and breath to the center of your chest (your heart center). Imagine every time you allow a breath into the body you are warming your heart center, and every time you release your breath, tension is released. See if you can sense if you are pressing your heart center down, back, or pushing it forward. See if you can soften your heart center and allow it to relax and float up and over your belly, without pushing or holding it up.

7   *Spine:* Bring your attention to your tailbone. With your mind's eye trace up your spine, imagining little pockets of air between each of your 26 vertebrae — again, without pulling up. Bounce your knees slightly to make sure you are allowing the bones of your legs to support you. Do not forget your neck and the topmost vertebra, which is close to the center of your head.

8   *Head:* Bring your attention to your head. See if you can sense if you are pushing your chin up or down, or straining upward with your head. Imagine your head simply floating on top of your spine. Relax your tongue in your mouth. Allow your jaw to relax, and breathe through your mouth.

9   Imagine your weight pouring down into the floor through the bottom of your feet. Imagine your spine blooming up out of the floor. Sense your entire skeletal system, like the scaffolding of a house. Feel how sturdy the floor is under your feet. The more you allow your bones and the floor to support you, the more your spine can bloom up out of the floor. Imagine every time the breath releases out of the body, you are releasing excess tension.

10 Press your feet down slightly into the floor with a sense of the bones blooming up from the floor. With your mind's eye, scan your body to see if you can sense if you are holding excess tension anywhere. Relax your face, eyes and tongue. Open your eyes and let your vision rest on whatever is in your line of sight. Breathe. We take the world in as we breathe in, and release energy out into the world as the breath is released out of the body.

For many, this type of self-observation exercise is completely new. In introductory courses when I ask students to notice what they are doing with their bodies their first impulse is to look for the wall mirrors in the studio. In other words, their way of noticing is by looking at the body as an object, separate from themselves. This exercise can be a first step to directing attention inwardly, listening, sensing and noticing the body.

I do *Standing Alignment* in every class. Repetition is essential to cultivate the ability to sense where you are holding excess tension, which areas of the body feel blocked or frozen, and where energy is not flowing freely. The more you initially work with eyes closed and employ the mind's eye to guide attention and breath to specific areas of the body, the deeper and more specific your sensory awareness and self-observation skills become. With this skill comes an ability to make subtle, micro-adjustments in the body.

It can take time to trust and understand that alignment is not a process of muscle manipulation. The more you allow the bones to support your weight, the more you will release excess muscular tension. The result is greater ease and grace in your movement. This is part of the process of initiating and re-patterning the flow of energy through the body's core.

Sequence 2: Centering

HANDS-ON CENTERING

We tend to hold tension in the belly, and in a culture that is preoccupied with thin physiques and having a flat tummy, it is an area we tend to suck in, hide, and pretend is not there. It is a powerful area of the body, and the seat of our emotions. Therefore, directing attention to the belly and lowering the center of gravity to this area can initially be disorienting. Some of my students report feeling a little dizzy while engaged in this exercise. This is common when there is a sudden release of excess tension or the body is reorganizing and reorienting to a new center of gravity. Working with eyes open can help alleviate any initial discomfort.

1   Begin with *Standing Alignment*. Place one hand on your lower belly, a few inches below your navel. Place the back of your other hand across the flat of your back, below the waist.

2   Close your eyes. With your mind's eye imagine your breath dropping into the space between the hand on the front of your body and the hand on your back. Try to release all your abdominal muscles. Continue to allow your breath to drop into your center.

3   Sense how much space there is between your two hands. Allow all that space to fill up with weight, warmth and energy. Take your time. If you start to feel dizzy, open your eyes.

4   Continuing to breath into your center, extend your attention from your center to the bottom of your feet. Imagine the weight in your center pouring through the center of the bones in your legs, through the bottom of your feet, down into the floor.

5   Keeping your feet planted on the floor, slowly move your center slightly forward. Notice more weight pouring into the balls of your feet. Move your center slightly back, and notice more weight pouring into your heels. Move your center to the right, and notice weight pouring out of one foot and more weight going into the other foot.

6 Now play with slowly circling your center, keeping your attention on the redistribution of weight on the bottom of your feet.

7 Bring your center back to center — feel your weight evenly distributed between your left and right foot, and on the tripod of your feet.

You can do this exercise and the following exercise, *Center Walks*, with a partner. One person has hands on their partner's center and lower back. Hands-on work helps guide attention. The person with hands-on needs to focus and breathe. If doing the following exercise with a partner, the person walking may keep their eyes closed the entire time. This may make it harder to balance while walking slowly, but can deepen one's sense of center and the ability to listen to the body.

CENTER WALKS

We all tend to rush — physically and mentally. Some parts of us seem to always be ahead or behind other parts of us — thinking, anticipating, calculating and focusing on an end goal. A component to centering is lining up all of these parts in the present moment. In other words, you align and center your energy and intention.

In this exercise you move extremely slowly. Slow motion gives you time to notice and sense the mechanics and dynamics of what you are doing and what is happening in the present moment. It encourages your brain to slow down and line up with the body. There is a noticeable shift when you entirely give over to slow motion. It's as if the brain finally surrenders its insistent on being in charge and running the show. There is a physical and energetic release, a uniformity of rhythm throughout the body and one's being, and an overall sense of ease when one entirely surrenders to slow motion.

This is a focused walk forward. Visualize pouring weight from your center into the floor through the feet as you exhale. The tendency to hold one's breath while focusing is common. Remember to breathe and to move very, very slowly. You are entering more of a geological rhythm and time frame, rather than a natural human rhythm and time frame.

1 Bend both of your knees slightly to lower your center of gravity. Move your center to the left until all of your weight is pouring through your left leg and into the floor through your left foot. As you do this, feel the weight slowly drain out of your right foot, until there is no more weight in your right foot.

2 Imagine fine sand pouring from your center through the bones of your legs, through the bottom of your feet, and down into the floor. See if you can allow your spine to keep blooming up, your heart center floating, and your head floating on the top of your spine as you do this.

3 Imagine a string attached to your right knee, and someone gently tugs the string forward. The heel of your right foot is now in contact with the floor slightly in front of you.

4 From your center, slowly begin to pour your weight into your right leg. Feel the weight going through the heel of your foot, then the outside of your foot, to the ball of your foot, until you are centered over the tripod of your right foot, and there is no weight in your left foot. Repeat. Release your breath as you release your weight into the floor.

I have witnessed monks in different cultures engaged in a slow, purposeful walk as a form of meditation. Once students have repeated this exercise a number of times, it becomes second nature, whether going slowly or walking at a normal pace. Many of my students use this exercise as a way to relax, get centered and focused before performing.

CENTER STRINGS

There is a tendency to lose our physical awareness and sense of center when we are in relationship to others. Just as jugglers begin to practice with two balls, add another, and then another, we do the same in many of these sequences of exercises. We begin with grounding our awareness in ourselves, and immediately extend it to include another. Remaining open to internal impulses and being responsive to others' energy and actions is necessary for the actor to establish believable relationships on stage.

In this exercise you practice extending awareness to include one other person, then to three other people. Pausing frequently and finding a sense of stillness will help you remain relaxed and centered. This is a lively exercise that incorporates spatial awareness, tempo and rhythm. So the balls in the air include: awareness of center, awareness of a partner, changing speeds, pausing, and spatial relationships. The more you relax and breathe, the easier it is to genuinely take in and respond to others.

1   Stand facing a partner. Imagine a string extending from your center to your partner's center. Just let your eyes rest on your partner's eyes when facing them. (Don't look at the imaginary string or your partner's center.)

2   This string connecting you may be taut, like a string, or stretchy like a rubber band. It can be very short or very long. If you turn your back to your partner, imagine the string extends through the flat of your back, and see if you can sense where your partner is and what they are doing.

3   Both of you are going to move any way you wish — slowly and quickly, sometimes moving at the same time, sometimes not. Pause often. You are always moving in response to each other, and always attached by this imaginary string. Breathe.

4   Move far away from your partner. Move very close to your partner. Change levels. Change speeds. Don't forget to interrupt your movement with moments of stillness.

5 After improvising for 5–10 minutes, pair up with another duo so you are now in a group of four. Stand in a circle. You now have three strings extending to the three people in your group. Start to move slowly. If you feel disconnected at any time, pause or slow your movement down. Work in your group for 5–10 minutes.

6 Now stand, and in your mind's eye cut the string. Walk around the room on your own.

It is possible to become highly tuned in to your partner in this exercise, which can produce a sense of joy and fun that comes with genuinely working in response to a partner. I often use this exercise as a warm-up into scene work and staging scenes with large groups. It produces noticeable results in actors' aliveness to each other and the space.

Centering and Alignment reinforces a balance between tension and release that is addressed in all of the exercises. A centered stillness is a balance between tension and release. There is a tendency to associate energy with excess tension, and relaxation with collapse.

In many Western practices, there is an association with the floor as the place to completely give into gravity. In many Eastern practices, the floor is perceived as the ground through which things extend upward. Think of plants that bear roots down into the earth in order to gain nourishment to sprout upwards towards the sun. In Sequences 1–3, we establish the floor as a source of support. Students learn to *pour weight* into the floor, then how to use the floor as a surface to *bloom up from*, and eventually how to *work off of* the floor.

Centering and Alignment need to be reinforced through repetition of these exercises combined with hands-on work, floor exercises, and consistent side coaching and reminders. No one exercise replaces a thorough training in techniques that address alignment, or physical, emotional and mental habits. These first sequences of exercises are intended to supplement and reinforce comprehensive work in these important areas of training, not just as a necessary prerequisite for movement work, but to establish an important ground of awareness.

Sequence 3: Moving from Center

STARFISH

This exercise involves initiating and moving from center while remaining released into the floor. The focus is on moving all five points of the "starfish" — head, arms, and legs, uniformly. The sense is of gathering the five points of the star around your center, and then extending out and away from center, while engaging as few muscles as possible. Ease, breath, and energy flowing uniformly through the core of the body through the extremities are key.

1   Lie on your back with your arms on the floor, extended at an angle over your head and legs spread, so you are making a big "X" on the floor. Breathe into your center.

2   Sense how your two arms, two legs and head are all radiating away from your center, like the five-points of a star.

3   Feel all the places your body is in contact with the floor. Take a moment to notice if there are places you are holding tension, and see if you can relax your muscles and bones into the floor.

4   Initiating from your center and remaining as relaxed as possible, begin to slowly *fold* your five points — head, arms and legs — around your center, to bring you into the fetal position on your side. Go slowly. Keep as many surfaces of your body in contact with the floor at all times, as if you were painting the floor with your body. Once you are in the fetal position, feel all the places your body is in contact with the floor. Release into the floor and breathe in this position.

5   Begin to *unfold* your five points away from your center to bring you onto your belly, in an "X" with arms over your head and legs apart. Again, stay as relaxed as possible. Imagine energy radiating from your center. Engage as few muscles as possible, and keep as many surfaces of your body in contact with the floor as possible. Once you are lying on your belly, scan your body to see if your weight is fully released into the floor. Breathe.

6 Repeat the folding to come into the fetal position on your other side.

7 Repeat the unfolding to come onto your back into your original "X" position.

8 Repeat this sequence one or two more times on your own. Go slowly. Breathe.

STANDING STARFISH

Once you have done *Starfish* on the floor, the challenge is to remain relaxed and to keep movements fluid while standing. You are initiating movement from your center and radiating energy from your center to the extremities. You are trying to move as a cohesive whole — spine, arms, legs, and head, moving in rhythm to the breath. This exercise encourages awareness and energy to uniformly move through the upper and lower halves of the body, the extremities and the spine simultaneously.

1 Stand in *Starfish* — a big "X" with legs about two feet apart, arms extended out and above your shoulders. Relax your shoulders into your back. Feel a little weight in your tailbone. Relax your rib cage. Allow the neck to be long and the head to float on top of your spine. Breathe. Again, sense how the five points of your star are all radiating away from your center.

2 Imagine energy and breath radiating from your center through your solar plexus and upper chest, through your arms and out all of your fingertips. Feel energy radiating from your center, up your spine and out the crown of your head, down your legs and into the floor through your feet.

3 Take a breath in, and as you release your breath you are going to gently fold the five points of your star around your center. At the same time, beginning at the tailbone, you are going to gently round your back, and bend your knees.

4 As you take a breath in, unfold, beginning from your center. When you come back to your starting position, do not over-extend by pushing your ribs and chest forward or your tailbone up or out. Keep it simple and easy.

5   All five points of your star are equally important. You are initiating this movement from your center — not your upper chest and shoulders. Keep you shoulders completely relaxed.

6   Continue to fold and unfold. Think of seaweed gently swaying back and forth to the pulse of the ocean. Keep your movements smooth and flowing.

7   Don't forget to bend your knees. Coordinate your breath, so you are folding for the duration of your exhale, and unfolding for the duration of your inhale.

Once you are familiar with the mechanics of this exercise, introduce imagery: breathe in and out like gentle waves and the ebb and flow of the sea. You are like seaweed, gently folding and unfolding in the water.

For many, coordinating the pelvis, knees, and spine in this exercise takes time. As our attention is often on our thoughts, there tends to be more energy in the head, neck, and shoulders than the spine and lower half of the body. Keep an eye out for the tendency to initiate unfolding with the upper chest, neck, and shoulders instead of from the center and spine. Remember to bend the knees, and to not over-effort and over-extend by pushing the ribs forward or arching the back when unfolding to standing.

MOVING CENTER

We tend to engage the head, neck and shoulders in almost all actions, from simply sitting down to standing up. Our legs are sorely
underused. In this exercise, you press down through your legs to
work *off of* the floor. The quality of pressing the knee to bend the
leg has more energy and tension in it, and is more bound than just
bending the knee.

1   Begin standing with your legs about two feet apart. With a sense
of your center, press and bend your right knee, and feel your
center move to the right. Feel your weight pouring into the floor
through your right foot.

2   Instead of straightening your leg by pushing your knee back,
gently press down into the floor through your right foot so your
leg straightens. You are pressing down into the floor to move
your center from side to side. Repeat this to the other side. Now
repeat this from side to side.

3   Keep your spine and head easy and radiating up from your center.
Your body is just going along for the ride that your legs are
providing. Your legs are doing the work here.

4   Now bring one leg about two feet in front of you. Repeat this
exercise, moving front to back. Again, just press and bend one
knee at a time, and sense your center moving forward and back.

5   Continuing to engage your legs, keeping your attention on your
center, you are now going to take your center for a ride through
the space. Begin to move through the room, pressing and
bending the knees. Now when you straighten your legs, gently
press down into the floor to push off of the floor. It is similar to
a little jump, and one foot may come off the floor. Stay centered
over both your legs. Turn, move backward and forward. Keep
your spine, head and shoulders easy. They are just "going along
for the ride." Keep bending those knees. Breathe.

Sequence 4: Sharing Center

There is a day care center near my home. At the end of the day the two- and three-year olds wait in the playground for their parents to pick them up. I saw one child standing very still in the middle of the playground. When he saw his mother approaching down the street, a huge smile emerged on his face. He started to make sounds, flapped his arms, and jumped up and down. He was literally bouncing with joy to see his mother.

We learn to stifle our natural responses as we grow up. And as we grow, more tension gets stored in the body, which masks sensation. This limits the level of our responsiveness and emotional/ physical flexibility. An open and highly responsive body, alive to impulse, is essential for the actor. In order to establish believable relationships on stage the actor's body must become sensitive and agile enough to respond quickly to moment-to-moment internal shifts and external stimuli.

In the following sequence you work in direct response to a partner, first receiving information and responding through touch and physical contact. These exercises are inspired by Contact Improvisation, an improvisational movement form that involves a physical dialogue between two or more people — weight-sharing, counterweight, momentum, lifts, falls, and rolls.

BACK TO BACK

Working in partners, sit on the floor with either your legs crossed or knees bent with feet on the floor, or any position that is comfortable where your spine can be long. Sit with your back in contact with a partner. Adjust so you have as much of your back in contact with your partner's back as possible, without straining.

1 Close your eyes. Begin to breathe into your back. Feel the surfaces of your back in contact with your partner. See if you can put breath in your back, so your partner feels the subtle expansion of your spine and ribs as you breathe, and visa versa. Just use your

breath to create subtle movement and connection between you and your partner's back.

2 Now begin to move a little more, keeping the movement slow. Expand up your spine, gently press one rib back, slowly undulate your spine, subtly roll from side to side along your rib cage, move one shoulder blade, press through your lower back. See how subtly and specifically you can make your movements. Move very slowly. You are moving together, as if you had one spine between you. You are both initiating and following.

3 Occasionally bring the back of your heads into contact, and the backs of your arms.

4 Begin to move a little more, and give a little more of your weight to your partner. Lean into your partner's back, so they fold forward, and vica versa.

5 Now slowly begin to decrease the movement, so again, you are just breathing into each other's backs, through your backs. The movement is subtle.

6 Come to stillness, open your eyes, and fold forward, to peel your backs away from each other.

Do this for 5–10 minutes. At the end of this exercise you can experiment with coming to a standing position sharing weight with your partner:

7 Sit back-to-back with a partner, knees bent, feet on the floor and close to your body.

8 Begin to gently pour your weight through your lower, mid and upper back into your partner's back. Do this incrementally, so you and your partner are pressing into each other's backs with the same amount of weight.

9 When you feel a strong sense of contact with your partner begin to press into the floor through your feet as you continue to press into your partner's back, to come to a standing position together, backs in contact. This should be a smooth and relaxed movement together to come to standing. Breathe as you rise to your feet.

COUNTERWEIGHT

Counterweight and weight-sharing exercises reinforce a sense of one's center and moving from center. Individual guidance and side coaching is useful when teaching this exercise to help actors pour their weight and work from center versus over-engaging their arm and shoulder muscles.

1 Standing in alignment, slowly begin to round your back. Bend your knees. The impulse begins at the tailbone rounding under, and gently pressing back through your ribs and spine. Gently round your back and allow the head to fall forward. Relax your shoulders, gently pressing your scapula down.

2 Continuing to press back through the spine and ribs. Now pour your weight from your center behind you so you begin to fall backwards. You will have to take a few steps backwards so you don't fall down. Repeat this a few times.

3 You are going to repeat this, but now you are going to do it with a partner. This time your feet won't move to keep you from falling — you will be holding your partner's hands in a counterweight balance.

4 Face a partner and stand about two feet apart. With relaxed arms place your hands on each other's wrists.

5 Both of you will bend your knees and round your backs. Very slowly begin to pour your weight directly behind you. As you do this, your arms will slowly begin to straighten and you will feel increasing pressure where you two are holding hands. You are keeping each other from falling backwards. This is counterbalance.

6 To come back to a standing position facing your partner, your brain is going to tell you to pull in with your arm and shoulder muscles. Instead, take a breath, bend the arms slightly and bring your center back over your own two feet as you take a breath. This will prevent putting excess tension in your arms and shoulders.

After you become accustomed to pouring weight in counterbalance with a partner, there are endless ways to explore: standing side-by-side holding hands and leaning away from each other; standing in a circle of four or more holding hands and leaning back; and getting up from and down to the floor using counterweight and weight-sharing with a partner, either back to back or in this set-up of holding hands facing each other.

COMPLETE AGREEMENT

This is a leading-and-following exercise in light contact. Central to this exercise is staying connected to a sense of your center while in direct contact with another person, offering no resistance while following and having clear intention while leading. As you progressively tune into your partner, the sense is of the movement occurring between you, or both participants simultaneously leading and following.

1   Stand and face a partner, about 3 feet apart. Take a moment to come into *Standing Alignment*. Breathe and rest your eyes on your partner's eyes. Find the balance between looking at and taking in your partner, and let some of your attention drop to your center.

2   Spreading your fingers a bit, raise your hands and press your fingertips gently into your partners' fingertips. In your minds eye, connect your arms to your back and your center. See if you can relax your arms and hands a bit, but still have energy in them.

3   One of you will initiate and one of you will respond. As the responder, you are not passively letting your partner move your arms around. Both of you have energy in your hands and arms and are gently pressing into each other's fingertips.

4   As the initiator, move your hands slowly, and pause from time to time. Your hands are initiating, but they move your torso and head. Change levels, twist, reach and pause. Move very slowly and smoothly. Keep your hands and arms connected to your center, and stay in eye contact.

5 You should not be able to tell who is initiating and who is following. Continue to relax, breathe into your center, and don't over-concentrate.

6 Without stopping, switch who is initiating. Move slowly.

7 Switch who is initiating again.

8 Now both of you lead and both of you follow. If you feel connected to your partner, you can begin to move through space. Go slowly and continue to interrupt the movement with moments of stillness.

This is a wonderful exercise to lead into any kind of scene work. It is also a good lead-in to any kind of partner dancing. I often give the instruction every one or two minutes to switch who is initiating. This may happen four or five times before I tell students to both lead and follow (#8). As actors drop into this exercise, thinking, self-consciousness and worry tend to be replaced with the pleasure and ease that comes with feeling connected to, and completely joining another person in an activity. Instead of the tension that may accompany a sense of having *to do something* or achieving a specific result, you can relax into a sense of *lending oneself* to an activity.

This attitude, sense and skill are key components to all of these exercises, and to approaching text and scene work. Similar to the *Authentic Movement* process (Part Two), actors begin to potentially experience the difference between moving and allowing oneself to be moved. There is a distinct difference between imposing one's thoughts and ideas on a piece of text, and exploring speaking a piece of text to discover what thoughts, feelings, instincts, impulses and associations are inspired in the moment of speaking. In other words, *allowing the text to work on you*. We will explore this in more detail in the last two sections of this manual.

Sequence 5: Radiating from Center

Expand and Fold furthers the distinction between tension and energy. In this sequence you specifically direct and project your energy beyond the body. The focus is less on the mechanics of the movement (as in *Starfish*) and more on the intention and motivation behind the movement. The final shapes you embody and how you get there are improvised and informed by your internal state, which is inspired by the image and sense of expanding and folding. In other words, instead of directing the movement, you are filling yourself with an intention, noticing, and following how the body responds.

EXPAND AND FOLD

1   Bring your awareness to the center of your body. Very slowly fill and expand the core of your body with your breath and energy — beginning in the lower belly, to the solar plexus, to the center of the chest — filling your core like you are filling a glass with warm water.

2   Once your core feels filled, allow this expansion to radiate out to the surfaces of your body. Take your time. Allow the energy to expand down your legs, through your arms and fingers, up your spine into your head and eyes. Allow this energy to animate the body, with the sense that your energy is expanding past the surfaces of your body and out into the room. You are going to expand out and up on a diagonal, as if you are reaching for something you really want but that is just out of reach. Do not push or put excessive tension in your muscles. See if you can find a full sense of expansion, without constricting or locking your muscles. Just sense energy radiating from your core, through your body out into the room.

3   Move very slowly and notice what is happening as you begin to move. In other words, don't focus on the end point but turn your focus on your movement, breath and internal sense or inner states along the way.

4   Very, very slowly begin to drain this energy out of the body. Reverse the process, so you begin to incrementally bring your energy back towards your body, then to your extremities, to the surfaces of your body and into your core. Go past your starting position/state (neutral) and allow your body to fold in and down. Folding in has a softer, gentler quality than *contracting* or *collapsing*.

Go very slowly and keep breathing. The goal is not to reach an end position but to keep noticing inner states and the body moving along the way to the two end points of expanding out and folding in and down. The quality of attention in this exercise tends to be riveting. In a classroom setting, after actors have explored on their own I divide the group in half to watch. This helps actors see and begin to trust the powerful expressive potential of movement when there is clear focus and intention.

SIX DIRECTIONS

Using *Expand and Fold*, you will now focus on different directions — front, back, above, below, and to the sides. You can either notice what images, senses or feelings arise as you engage in this exercise, or you can begin by employing imagery.

Our attention tends to orient towards goals or the culmination of an action. And we tend to focus on the external action rather than the internal experience of and motivation behind an action. There is meaning in our choice of actions, but there is also content in *how* we engage in an action.

In this exercise you are moving slowly enough to notice and track your subtle, internal, ever-changing energetic dynamics. When teaching this exercise, I often provide a variety of images that engage many senses and inspire different intentions. Music can add to the power of this exercise. Following is an example of the types of images I employ:

1   *Expand above:* Imagine you feel a warm ray of sunlight on your forehead. It radiates down through your lower back and belly, through your legs, up your spine, into your heart, across your shoulders, and up into your face. Slowly begin to reach up towards the sun. Once you feel filled with warmth and light, slowly begin to fold.

2   *Expand on the sides:* You smell the scent of a sweet apple. You are very hungry. Imagine you have never smelled that scent before or seen an apple. Breathe the scent into your belly as you expand. Slowly look up and to your side. You see a big red apple hanging from a branch of a tree. Continuing to expand, reach up towards it. Once you pick the apple, begin to slowly fold, bringing the apple towards your center.

3   *Expand behind:* You hear the voice of someone dear to you that you have not seen for a very long time. Breathe in the sound of their voice — into your belly, solar plexus and heart. Very slowly begin to twist to look behind you. You see them. You reach for them. As you reach for them their image fades. Begin to fold away.

4   *Below:* You see a very small and beautiful bird on the ground in front of you. Very slowly begin to reach down towards it. As you get closer to it, it flies into your hand. Fold.

EXPAND AND FOLD WITH A PARTNER

In this exercise you track your inner sensations and responses that arise from the physical experience of expanding and moving, with the additional focus of working with a partner.

1 Face a partner and stand about five feet apart. Begin in *Standing Alignment*. Allow your eyes to rest on your partner's eyes. Breathe.

2 Very slowly both of you will begin to expand towards each other. Once you have expanded out towards your partner, slowly begin to fold away from each other. Notice again that you pass through your starting position on your way to folding in and away from your partner.

3 Now, Partner A begins to expand towards Partner B, and Partner B begins to fold away. Partner A initiates the action and Partner B is folding away *in response* to A.

4 Once Partner A is completely expanded and Partner B is completely folded, Partner B begins to expand toward Partner A. Now Partner A begins to fold *in response* to Partner B.

5 Repeat. Move slowly and keep noticing what you are sensing and feeling. Take your cues off each other and move in response to each other.

The experience of directly expanding energy and movement from our centers to another person — or folding energy away from another — is physical, energetic, and psychological. If working in a group, divide the group in half to watch partners after they have explored on their own.

Sequence 6: Actor and Audience

In the *Expand and Fold* exercises you radiate your energy outward starting at your core, and this expansion animates the body. In this exercise you are going to remain in the *Standing Starfish* position (the "X:" arms extended up, legs apart). The expansion changes the quality of your energy and presence while you remain still, in a slightly suspended state. You will then extend your awareness in the following exercise, *The Village*, to include an audience.

EXPAND IN STILLNESS

1   Begin in a standing *Starfish* — legs apart, arms extended up and to the diagonals, your body in a big "X."

2   Without changing this position, begin the process of expanding — starting at the core, radiating to the surfaces of the body, out to the extremities, into the room and now past the walls, floor and ceiling of the room. You are simultaneously radiating behind through your back, above through the crown of your head, to the front, sides and diagonals. Breathe.

3   See of you can relax your attention enough to expand your awareness in all directions. Do not push. Allow your breath to drop into your center and radiate your energy out into the room as you exhale.

4   Now begin to bring your energy and attention back in a bit to the surfaces of your body. Release your arms down and bring your feet underneath your hip sockets to come into *Standing Alignment*.

Images can be useful in this exercise to get energy moving throughout the body. You can imagine a ball of light in the center of the body, light beams radiating through the arms and out of each fingertip, shining out of the heart center into the room and through all the surfaces of your back behind you, up the spine, and out of the forehead, eyes, and crown of the head, down into the floor through the bottom of the feet. Visualize the light beams illuminating the whole room, and even going past the walls and ceiling. The key is to stay relaxed in a state of expansion. See if you can identify the moment you may begin to over-effort, or begin to constrict your energy. When you bring your energy back in, imagine you are surrounded by a luminous ball of light radiating from all surfaces of the body — out of every pore and cell.

THE MOUNTAIN

This exercise encourages coming into your natural alignment while moving and radiating energy out to the edges of your personal space, or *kinesphere*. The more you practices this, the more you can "be in your mountain" effortlessly. Many of my former students, years after graduating, have reported utilizing this exercise in their daily lives and professional work.

1 Come into *Standing Alignment*.

2 Imagine a luminous, permeable cone of light surrounding you. We will call this your *mountain*. It is your *kinesphere*, or personal space. It extends above the crown of your head, behind you, in front of you, to your sides, and down to the floor. Use your extended arms to trace the dimension of your mountain in all directions.

3 Making small, circular motions with your hands, holding your arms straight, "wash" the inside surfaces of your mountain in all directions.

4 With the sense of standing in the center of your mountain, expand your energy and attention to its surfaces — above the crown of your head, in front of you, behind your back, from your ribs out to your sides, around your legs and down to the floor.

5 Keeping your eyes on the horizon, turn 360 degrees. Try not to blink, and try to relax your awareness to all the surfaces of your mountain as you turn.

6 Now walk around the room with the sense of taking your mountain for a walk. Keep your awareness extending above, behind, to the sides and front. Notice others, and respect the dimensions of their mountains. See if you can do this with a sense of ease.

The Mountain is just a sense — you don't have to "do" anything. The more you relax and breathe into your center, the more you have the potential to effortlessly expand your energy and awareness.

THE VILLAGE

The purpose of this exercise is to practice remaining centered and relaxed while taking in an audience. This practice promotes an open and available presence as opposed to the constricted and defensive presence that audition and performance anxiety can illicit. This exercise also provides an opportunity to observe your own and other's habits — the ways in which we manifest tension and deflect energy, such as holding our breath, fidgeting, sinking into one hip, smiling, or putting on a social mask. Standing and not producing material, or "doing nothing" is intimate, and can initially make students uncomfortable.

This exercise can be an introduction to performing in front of the class or an audience. It involves seeing and inviting to be seen, experiencing and being experienced. It is also an introduction to how to watch each other's work in a classroom setting. It requires active listening: students watching are sitting up, breathing, and bringing their full attention to the performer at all times in this — and every presentation in class that has an audience component.

This is a solo exercise with an audience component. I often set up the exercise this way: The ancient, traditional view of the performer is that they are the vehicles through which the energy of the earth and heavens reveal themselves. You have been invited by your village (your classmates, in this case) to be the vessel through which we all engage for this moment. It is an honor and an indication of your graciousness and generosity to accept the invitation.

You enter the performance space *as an observer*, and you are in an exchange with your village. You are with them, they are with you, and it is a simple, human exchange.

1 Begin in *Standing Alignment* and establish *The Mountain*.

2 Enter the space and face your village. Breathe and center yourself. Feel the floor underneath you.

3 Allow your eyes to graze on the eyes of your audience, one at a time, as you breathe and take them in. This is done fairly quickly, and does not need to be heavy or overly significant. Just take your audience in. Keep your *Mountain* active, and breathe.

4 Turn 360 degrees, with the sense of being in the center of your mountain. Keep your eyes on the horizon, and take in what you see as you turn.

5 Face your audience again, turn and exit. In your minds eye and awareness, take the audience with you.

I have auditioned numerous people for theater productions and entrance into acting programs. It is common for young actors to either pull their energy in and down, or turn their backs to their auditors to focus themselves before beginning the audition. Usually, they appear quite tense as they do this, as if they were girding themselves for a dangerous solo feat. The stakes are high, but auditioning is a human exchange. What a difference it makes when actors enter the room in a centered and relaxed state, and begin their work by taking in their auditors simply, and breathing for a moment. After practicing *The Mountain* and *The Village*, these exercises can be done quickly in preparation for an audition or before walking on stage. These exercises help cultivate an inviting, generous and confident stage presence before the first words of a monologue are spoken. The effect is stunning.

PART TWO

The Intuitive Body

Do you have the patience to wait
till your mind settles and the water is clear?
Can you remain unmoving
until the right action arises by itself?

— Tao Te Ching

Sequence 1: Movement In Depth

In this sequence you will begin with an inner-directed focus. You then expand awareness to include the environment, to working in response to images and other people. The first exercise is a meditative, self-directed process based on one aspect of *Authentic Movement*. Originally called *Movement-In-Depth* by its founder, Mary Starks Whitehouse, *Authentic Movement* grew out of her work in modern dance, dance improvisation, dance/movement therapy, and her work with the psychiatrist Carl Jung in *Active Imagination*. *Authentic Movement* is applied within psychotherapeutic frameworks, and it is also a creative process utilized by artists and performers.

Authentic Movement is the practice of quieting mental activity enough to listen and give form through movement to the river of sensations, impulses, images, feelings and memories that runs through all of us all of the time. We gain access to this river — the source of all of our imaginative impulses — through the body. Through this process, actors become more sensitive to the nature of impulse and how to notice, experience and respond to impulses as they arise from moment to moment.

The form of *Authentic Movement* is very simple. Students move with eyes closed while being witnessed. This is not a performance method — it is a movement *process*. It allows us to notice and give form to genuine internal impulses without having to focus on or worry about performance or presentation. Many students, free from direction or choreography, discover a wider range of movement, and are surprised by the pleasure and depth of their experience.

The body tends to have a lot to say when we simply listen and get out of our own way. A variety of material and experiences arises in this work, from the simple joy of consciously moving, to a range of emotions, memories, and personal, psychological material. I reassure students that whatever arises is appropriate. Just notice and respond.

This moment-to-moment following the body's lead involves simultaneously moving and *allowing oneself to be moved*. It requires a delicate balance between will and surrender. Finding and maintaining this balance can be trained like a muscle. The concept of surrender has many associations such as passivity, giving up, or giving over to the will of another. In this context it is an ability to give over to something other than one's thoughts, fears, perceptions — to fully *lend oneself to something* — body, mind, and spirit. This *surrendering* takes courage, devotion, and a lot of practice. It is an essential aspect of the ability to remain embodied, available, and responsive to and in the present moment — on stage, while speaking and while responding to another. This is the key component of the quality of attention that inspires a compelling immediacy and vitality to our presence and our work on stage.

So much of actor training is designed to guide students past the obstacles and habits of thinking and perception that prevent them from accessing the full depth and range of their genuine experience. As simple as this form is, the practice of Authentic Movement can be challenging. The skills gained in Authentic Movement are subtle, but they can have a profound impact on an actor's development.

Moving with the eyes closed often frees students from the experience of the body as object, worrying about what they look like, judging their choices or physical ability. The tendency to judge and categorize experiences is common, and this potentially limits choices. Judgment is like a big foot that steps on the imagination. Most of us have ongoing loops of less than useful thoughts. As the actor's instrument is him/herself, they are particularly susceptible to the habit of self-criticism. This movement process can help actors notice their internal judges and dialogue, which is the first step to coming into a healthier relationship to both. Actors eventually learn how to suspend judgment, and in doing so, activate the imagination and gain access to a fuller emotional range.

When emotions arise they often grab all of our attention. We tend to attach to them — hook, line, and sinker, which potentially takes us out of the present moment and diminishes our physical awareness. Emotional agility is an ability to access a range of emotions and to allow them to inform us and move through us, without attaching meaning or labels or getting stuck in content or story. The root of the word "emotion" is "motion." Emotions *move through* us.

When facilitating this process, I wait until there is a level of comfort and trust between students and myself before introducing this type of inner-directed process. How you set up this process makes all the difference in the depth of the students' experience. The following exercises are not to be done consecutively in one class, but over many classes. After actors are familiar with this process, it can be used as a warm-up to other exercises.

Although most facilitators of Authentic Movement have trained for numerous years in this practice, in its most basic form and in this context, I believe it is not only appropriate for movement teachers to introduce, it is a rich resource for students of acting. Setting up the work clearly, providing a safe and supportive atmosphere, and adhering to the format of the written and verbal component at the end of the exercise is important. As the teacher/facilitator, you are witnessing your students and tracking your own experience.

AUTHENTIC MOVEMENT

All day long, we are either moving unconsciously or imposing our will on the body — directing our movement, as when we jog or take a ballet class. This process is neither of those. For the next 10–20 minutes, you are going to *follow* your body's lead. See if you can relax your thinking and notice what the body has to say. Nothing that arises is insignificant — sensations, impulses, images, feelings, memories, or thoughts. Just notice and respond by allowing the body to move and express itself. There is no correct or incorrect way to do this work. It is simply a space and time to listen and notice, and to let your body move the way *it* wants to move. Tell your brain to take a little vacation.

If you find you are not moving at all or are sleepy, breathe and energize your body a little. If you find you are not moving and just thinking, focus on your breath, and bring your attention to any sensations in the body. Sensation will be your lead and guide in this process.

Keep your eyes closed. If you have a sudden impulse to run around the room, squint your eyes so you don't bump into anything or anyone. If you have a sudden impulse to swing your arms around, take a quick look to make sure you don't injure anyone. Whatever arises is appropriate and fine. We are just giving the body a little airtime to say what it has to say today.

1   Walk around the room and see if you can let your body lead you to where you want to be in this room. Once you find a location, figure out if you want to be on the floor, standing or sitting. Take your time.

2   Close your eyes and focus on your breath. Imagine on every exhalation you are releasing excess tension.

3   With your mind's eye begin to scan the surfaces of your body. Notice where your body is in contact with the floor, the temperature of the air, the feeling of your clothes on your skin.

4   Now scan inside of your body. Let your mind's eye travel where it wishes.

5   Allow your attention to rest on one specific place of sensation in or on the body. It may be the taste inside your mouth, a hair tickling your face, dryness in your throat, tightness in your chest, warmth in your belly, or a muscle in your leg.

6   Once you find a specific place of sensation, let your minds eye rest on it. Go into the details. Just breathe and notice the details.

7   Let that go, and repeat the process to let your minds eye rest on a new place of sensation.

8   Now allow your body to begin to move. See what that place of sensation has to say. It is just a starting place. You can let your attention go where it will.

Directly after the movement session, I sometimes take 5 minutes to write. In this practice we do automatic writing — put pen to paper and just let the words flow. In other words, you are not writing *about* your movement experience but *from* it, so your writing is potentially as vital as your movement experience.

This applies to speaking too: if working in a group or with just one mover and one witness, you may wish to either speak about your movement experience or share what you have written or drawn. When speaking, the mover always speaks first, the witness second, and you do not comment on what anyone has said, or get into conversations. I believe this creates an atmosphere of safety, and encourages one to speak more freely. Writing and talking can help process the movement experience, and hearing the range of experiences in the room can be useful.

When facilitating this work I initially tell students that if they come into contact with another person, to just move away, as it can distract and take them out of the inner-directed listening. After practicing this process a little, they have a choice. If they come into contact with someone they can choose to move with them. If someone comes into contact with them and they do not want contact, they can clearly move away to continue working on their own.

SNAPSHOTS

This exercise addresses internal and external stimuli coming together. You begin with eyes closed and focus on your internal landscape, and then gradually open your eyes, to take in and respond to the environment.

1   Repeat the *Authentic Movement* process. About half way through the movement time (10–20 minutes) you will open your eyes for just a quick moment, a blink, and breathe in whatever you see — images, shapes, textures, colors. It is like taking a snapshot.

2   Close your eyes again. Imagine the image, shape, texture, color is developing and deepening inside of you. You are like a piece of sensitive photo paper.

3 With this imprint, follow how the movement plays out. Take another snapshot, and repeat the process.

4 After repeating this a few times, continue to move, and keep your eyes open most of the time. Keep your focus soft, and your attention on your internal landscape as you begin to extend your awareness simultaneously to the environment.

Sequence 2: Image Tableaux

In the *Authentic Movement* exercise you respond to internal stimuli as it arises moment-to-moment. Images may arise from the movement process, and these images inform internal states, which in turn inform the movement. In the following exercise you will begin with a specific image. The image informs your movement choices and the dynamic quality of your movement. Both of these ways of working strengthen the connection between the senses, imagination, feelings, memories, thoughts and actions. This exercise is inspired by work that was first introduced to me by Susan Dibble at Shakespeare and Company.

Here, principles of *Expand and Fold*, *Authentic Movement*, and *Snapshots* are combined. You can begin with any image, word or phrase. You are creating three positions or shapes with the body. They are a still tableaux. Leading into this type of work from *Authentic Movement* can help you avoid any tendency to illustrate your *ideas* with movement, or to work imitatively. This exercise can help you experience and witness the communicative power of gesture and shape. It can be done in silence or to music. Here we begin with the word and image "Harmony".

IMAGE RESPONSE

1. Harmony is a word filled with a variety of meanings. It suggests a state of grace, balance and ease. You may begin with specific visual images in your mind's eye, or sounds, or just fill yourself with a sense of what harmony feels like to you.

2. You will work with your eyes closed and begin in *Standing Alignment*. Similar to the *Expand and Fold* exercise, you are going to breathe into your center, and now fill yourself up with a sense or image of harmony. Allow the energy that is inspired by this word to expand and radiate out to all of the surfaces of your body, including your face. Do not move until you feel full to bursting with a sense of harmony.

3. Begin to move slowly. You will not be moving across the floor, but you will engage your whole body, and may change levels in space.

4. Pause when you find yourself in a position or shape that pleases you — one that feels like it embodies a sense of harmony. Breathe in this pause and just be still a moment.

5. When you are ready, continue to move slowly, until you find yourself in a new position. Pause.

6. Repeat this a third time. Pause, and then come back to the *Standing Alignment*.

7. Repeat the entire exercise, this time with the opposite image and sense: "Chaos."

ANTITHESIS

1. Repeat *Image Response* again, but now work with eyes open.

2. You will find two different moments of stillness in shapes that express "chaos" and two that express "harmony."

DUETS AND QUARTETS

1 You will now pair up with a partner to repeat the process of moving slowly and pausing in two shapes that express chaos and two shapes that express harmony.

2 Working with eyes open with a partner, both of you will pause at the same time in a shape or position you find together. You are not mirroring each other's shapes, but creating your individual shape in relationship to your partner's.

3 Begin by filling yourself up with a sense and feeling of the word or image, and trust your partner is doing the same.

4 You are essentially doing what you were doing on your own, but now you are also including a partner in your awareness, so together you are finding these shapes. You can work in light physical contact with each other or not.

After you have done this exercise once with a partner, if working in a group you can divide the group to watch each other's duets. I suggest doing this exercise to music.

Applications

I have applied this process in a wide variety of contexts. It is a good ensemble-building exercise, and can be used as a means to explore major themes in a play, to help actors viscerally connect to the world of a play, develop characters, and connect to their characters relationships with each other.

If you are working on a monologue or play, you can begin with a word or image from your text, or a word that expresses a major theme in the monologue or play. It can be applied to work with character, beginning with a quality, characteristic, or dynamic that you associate with your character. It can provide you with a physical, exploratory process in which to integrate and synthesize what you intellectually understand from your research of a play or character — to allow time to more intuitively sense and feel your way through your experience moment-by-moment.

PART THREE

The Receptive Body

You breathe; new shapes appear,
and the music of a desire as widespread
as Spring begins to move like a great wagon.
Drive slowly.

— Rumi

In Parts One and Two, a body and mind that are more centered, alive, open and responsive to impulse are cultivated. Parts Three through Five are physical improvisation explorations that help establish a bridge between the physical work, sound, and language. As improvisational skills increase, actors continue to form the physical, emotional, and mental flexibility to negotiate in the present moment, to communicate spontaneously from that experience, and to remain open and embodied while doing so.

My approach to physical improvisation has been deeply influenced by my work and training in Action Theater™. I believe every acting program and the work on our stages would benefit from all of the theories and practices of Action Theater, outlined in *Action Theater: The Improvisation of Presence*, and *Action Theater: The Manual*, written by Ruth Zaporah, Action Theater's creator. As Ruth describes it: "Exercises isolate the components of action — time, space, shape, and energy — so they can be examined, experienced, and altered in order to expand the expressive range and palette. The work provides tools to examine perceptive and responsive processes, and address habits that limit the ability to remain embodied, engaged, and in the moment. Fundamental to the practice of Action Theater is an embodied presence in performance, where the experiencing of the body informs the content of the moment, from moment to moment."[3]

The following sequences based on this approach have been condensed, changed, combined with other methods, and reframed specifically for actors. Similar to the sequences in the previous sections, it is important to allow time at the end of these exercises for participants to share their observations, impressions, questions, insights, and challenges.

In these exercises, you continue to strengthen the connection between the senses, feelings, imagination, and action — now working more directly in relationship, and with added sensitivity to timing and rhythm.

---

[3] www.actiontheater.com

Sequence 1: Ensemble

WALKING AND STILLNESS

This is both a self-observation exercise and a group collaboration. I often begin workshops, courses and rehearsals with this exercise. It builds a sense of ensemble, sets the tone in terms of the level of attention, energy, play and awareness expected in our work together.

1   Walk around the room at a fairly fast pace. Change directions often as if you were a slightly erratic person, and use all of the space in the room.

2   Now, initiate your walk with your eyes. Push energy out of your eyes, as if your eyes were grabbing the world, hungry and curious. Notice the room, colors, shapes and each other. Lean into it. Go further. There is tension and effort in this.

3   Now put your eyes in the back of your head. Notice if your pace shifts. See what you see, but do not let any energy out of your eyes. Even look at each other, but keep your eyes in the back of your head. Think about things — what you had for breakfast, where you have to go after class. This is the quality of energy and awareness that we sometimes walk around with in public. It is, in fact, quite private.

4   Stop. Now look out of your eyes as if receiving and inviting in the world around you. Actually see and take in what you are seeing. Allow energy out of your eyes but don't push.

5   Walk. Breathe and see each other. Let your eyes rest on others' eyes as you pass each other. This is not a social interaction, but you are taking others in as you walk.

6   Stop. Close your eyes. Go through *Standing Alignment* (Part One: Sequence 1) starting with your feet and moving up through the body to the crown of the head.

7   Open your eyes and allow the light and whatever is in your vision to come into your body. Breathe in your surroundings.

Imagine you can see from your eyes and the center of your chest simultaneously. Allow whatever you see to imprint on you as if you were a piece of sensitive photographic paper, and allow whatever is in your vision to deepen and develop inside you.

8 Allow the breath to drop into your center, and your attention to rest in the rhythm of your breath. Feel the support of the floor underneath you. Imagine the surfaces of your body softening, your back opening. Just breathe. This is *stillness*. It is an open, awake and energetic state.

STILLNESS

1 Now walk again at a fairly brisk pace, allowing energy out your eyes without pushing, and breathe into your center. Keep the pace up and change directions quickly and often. See each other, and keep imagining the surfaces of the body soft and receptive as you walk briskly. Let your eyes graze on people as you pass them. Don't pretend you are not walking in this room with other people! See them. You do not have to smile or greet them as you pass. You just have to breathe and notice each other and the room around you. There is nothing to think about. Just participate in this simple activity of walking in this room with these people.

2 Now occasionally *interrupt* your walking with stillness. This is not *a freeze* — which is a frozen "stop action." Stillness is an open, relaxed and alert state. Just abruptly stop walking, bring your attention to your breath, feel your feet underneath you, and center yourself. See and take in what is in your line of vision.

3 After you have been still, suddenly interrupt your stillness with walking. An *interruption to an activity* is sharper and clearer than a decision to be still or to walk. Make it very clear — 100 percent of you is still when you are still, then 100 percent of you is walking when you are walking.

4 When you are in stillness, feel the other people walking in the room around you. When you are walking, be aware of the people who are still in the room.

5 Sometimes be still for a long time, sometimes for a brief moment, and walk for different lengths of time. Surprise yourself. Be still when you least expect it, and interrupt the stillness with walking when you least expect it.

GROUP MIND

1 Now as you walk open up your peripheral vision. See if you can extend your awareness to everyone in the room, but keep your attention relaxed. When one of you interrupts the walking with stillness, all of you will be still. When one of you interrupts the stillness with walking, you all walk.

2 Do not anticipate action. Keep your attention relaxed. Be still longer than you expect or want.

3 Notice if you are the one always initiating the walking or stillness and let someone else initiate it. Breathe.

SHAPE/STATES

1 Instead of just standing in stillness, you are going to throw yourself into a melodramatic shape. You will be in a still tableau. This shape reflects a full-bodied inner state. Melodrama is an extreme state. It is not "kind of fond" — it is "madly in love." it is not "a little sad" — it is "grief ridden." it is not "sort of mad" — it is "filled with rage." it is not "kind of happy" — it is "bursting with joy." There is tension in melodrama. But see if you can continue to find the ground of stillness within that state. Breathe and fully inhabit wherever you are. Your face and eyes are part of it. It is not an empty shape — it is filled with feeling. Can you fully inhabit the full size and scope of melodrama, still breathe, and connect to a sense of stillness and the ground of inner calm?

2   You are still taking your timing from the group, so you will walk at the same time, and inhabit these still, melodramatic shapes and inner states at the same time. Retain that quality of interrupting your stillness with walking and vice versa. Deepen into it, breathe, and simply inhabit the temporary world of your shape/state. Do not plan. You do not have to know what you are doing. Just throw yourself into a shape, surprise yourself, and go to extremes.

3   Now every time you interrupt your walking with a melodramatic shape, add a sound.

4   When you throw yourself into melodramatic stillness, have it be in relationship or in response to others, without making physical contact.

5   Do not plan what you are going to do next. If you are planning, you are not in the experience of walking and being with each other. Simply throw yourself into a shape. See if you can become thoroughly saturated in whatever inner state the shape inspires in you.

6   If you notice you have not initiated a melodramatic stillness yet, do so. If you notice you are often initiating the walking, wait.

When teaching this work, I side-coach throughout this exercise. I often stop actors halfway through this part of the sequence to encourage them to go further and to get out of their comfort zone. There is tension in holding back energy. If you encourage actors to lend themselves completely to an activity and give them permission to let go and go further, they do. The result is deepened engagement; the level of play and energy in the room increases.

3-PART TABLEAUX

1   Walk. One person initiates a melodramatic shape. Then, the other members of the ensemble respond with their own melodramatic shapes. The ensemble remains still until someone initiates a new and dramatically different shape. Again, the other ensemble members respond with their own melodramatic shapes. Repeat this a third time, and after the last melodramatic shape and stillness, the group walks.

2   When throwing yourself into a melodramatic shape, respond to each other, so you are somehow engaged in the same "scene" while still moving into your own shapes and inner states.

3   Keep changing the duration of time you walk, and the duration of time you are all in a melodramatic stillness. Sometimes hold the stillness for a long time, sometimes just a moment.

The level of listening and response at the end of this exercise is usually quite remarkable. It can be a visceral experience of ensemble mind — of collaborating and being part of a highly tuned collective. Actors report feeling the moment the group relaxes, engages and starts to tune into and work together. This exercise tends to focus and energize the group, alleviate initial self-consciousness, and invites actors to experience working in ensemble.

Sequence 2: Initiation and Response

INITIATIONS THROUGH SPACE

In this warm-up you initiate movement with specific body parts. Remember the sense of following the body's impulses in the *Authentic Movement* process (Part Two). Instead of planning and controlling your movement, see if you can surprise yourself — allow the body to respond and not plan or think about your choices. This warm-up is lively, gets you moving through space, and incorporates rhythm, tempo, and momentum.

1   Imagine your brain leaves your head and travels to your knees. You are going to move in any way that your knees guide you to move. Initiate movement with your knees, and the rest of your body goes along for the ride. It's as if your knees had a mind of their own, and you are just following along. Move quickly, slowly, smoothly, percussively. Interrupt your movement frequently with long and short pauses.

2   Now your brain travels to your shoulders. Your shoulders have a mind of their own. Initiate a variety of movement with your shoulders. Remember to include moving through space.

3   Now your brain moves to your tailbone, pelvis and hips. Spiral, turn, jump. Make sure all your movements are initiated from this area and the rest of your body is following.

4   Don't forget to change speeds and occasionally interrupt your movement with moments of stillness.

5   Now your brain moves to your hands and your feet. You have four initiation points.

6   Now it moves to your head. Move slowly and pause more often, as you can get dizzy initiating with your head. Initiate from your eyelashes. Now your earlobe. Now the crown of your head. Don't forget to pause.

7　Continue to move on your own, pause, and change speeds, but now you decide which body part initiates. You can change initiation points whenever you wish. Try working with more than one initiation point — like your shoulders and knees, lips and belly.

Working with specific images and intentions for each body part in this exercise encourages moving in new ways and with varying dynamics. You can work with images such as: Imagine that your nose, eyes, ears, and mouth are in your knees. Your knees are very curious and want to explore the world. Then initiate with: sultry or seductive shoulders, shy feet, greedy belly, mischievous hips, proud elbows, innocent eyelashes, erratic hands, etc.

We tend to fall into repetitive patterns and rhythms when moving. Changing rhythms, dynamics, and pausing in stillness help us stay conscious and embodied. Remember that a pause is not a freeze, a moment to drop out of the present moment, or to think. It is a moment when external action is interrupted and suspended, but you are still saturated with your internal state. Pausing is an element in almost every exercise. It is a moment to notice and listen to your partner, yourself, and to deepen into the moment.

DEGREES OF RESPONSE

In this exercise you will work with a partner, playing with the degree and intensity of your responses. We are creatures of imitation. We tend to unconsciously match each other's behavior, energy level and dynamics. This can be deadly on stage. There is wonderful tension in contrast.

Part I

Working in partners, one of you will be the Initiator, the other the Responder.

INITIATOR

1   In the role of the Initiator, you will physically touch your partner to initiate movement. Keep your touch clear and consistent in terms of pressure and dynamic. You can use your hands and different body parts to initiate. For instance, use your knee to initiate behind your partner's knee, or use your shoulder to initiate on their back.

2   Once you have initiated an action on a specific part of your partner's body, follow your partner wherever they go. Stay interested in how they play out the initiation, as if you were highly fascinated by every detail of their response. Shadow their movements, levels and energy.

3   Let your partner come to stillness before you initiate again.

RESPONDER

1   In the role of the Responder you are going to play with the degrees of your response to your partner's initiations. If I were to assign a number between 0 and 100 to the energy with which we tend to respond to each other, it would probably be around 30. In this exercise you get to decide the degree of your response — anywhere from 0–100.

2   A "0" response means you hardly budge when your partner touches you. See what this feels like. A "100" response means you may move for quite a long time, and/or with lots of energy, speed or dynamism. In other words, you over-respond.

3   Begin your movement with the body part that has been touched by the Initiator, and move through space in the direction the initiation suggests.

4   You will come to stillness when that initiation point has played out, and then your partner will initiate again.

5   Each time you respond, do so at a different level — 10, 80, 50, 20, 100, etc. After about 5 minutes, switch roles.

In this exercise you can tune into your habit of response. If your tendency is to push or muscle responses, the lower levels of response (0–30) are useful. If you tend to lack energy or tend to play it cool or safe, the higher levels of response are useful.

In scene work, I notice beginning actors who are not speaking tend to drop out, or leave the present moment into the privacy of their thoughts. This exercise encourages active listening — a sustained level of focus and engagement from the person in the supporting role, the initiator in this case.

Part II

1 You will take this exercise into a more fluid duet. You will take turns physically initiating on each other.

2 Partner A will physically initiate Partner B. After Partner B has played out their movement, they will immediately physically initiate Partner A.

3 Each time your partner physically initiates, you will respond anywhere from 0–100. Use different body parts to initiate movement on each other.

4 As the initiator, stay engaged in the action and close to your partner as they play out that initiation.

INTERRUPTIONS WITH A PARTNER

In this exercise your attention is on form — time, shape, space, and rhythm. You are working with impulse in direct response to your partner. Focusing on form helps you stay tuned into the body from moment-to-moment as content — emotions, interpersonal dynamics, characters, or scenarios — arise out of your physical exchange. Content arising is appropriate, yet you want to also stay tuned to the form of your actions from moment-to-moment, rather than playing out a scenario.

1   Working with a partner, only one of you will move at a time. You will move until your partner interrupts you by moving. When you are interrupted, pause in whatever shape and inner state you are in. Breathe, notice and take in your partner. You are making offers to each other and are communicating to each other. You are always moving in response to your partner.

2   You may continue to work with body initiations, but you are now initiating yourself and are not in physical contact with your partner. You can initiate with one body part for a while, or change your initiation points quickly.

3   Sometimes contrast the rhythm and dynamics of what your partner was just doing. Sometimes interrupt your partner quickly, or sometimes let them go on for a while. In the pause, do not go away or think — instead breathe and notice your partner in whatever shape and inner state you were in when you were interrupted.

4   The more you focus on your partner you will intuitively know when you want to interrupt them. The second you have an impulse indulge it and interrupt them!

5   Change your spatial relationship. Sometimes move far away from each other. Sometimes move very close to each other. Change level, speed, tension level, and energy.

6   See if you can really take your partner in when they are moving, without worrying, thinking, or planning. Become fascinated with what they are doing.

When engaged in this exercise, make generous offers to each other — clear, bold choices as you are moving. When you are in a pause, breathe and take in what your partner is doing.

Exercises that sensitize actors to each other, increase their levels of responsiveness, and help them come genuinely into relationship to each other in their work are extremely important. Many of my students are fairly skilled at producing responses they imagine one would have if they were actually listening and being affected by their partner's actions. They are encouraged to deepen into these kinds of exercises to authentically experience their impact on their partner and to allow their partner to affect them. If you are thinking or planning, you are not available in the present moment — you are alone with your thoughts and plans. Once you come into relationship with your partner, the two of you respond genuinely to each other and the energy between you in this exercise will be palpable!

PART FOUR

The Speaking Body

How the flowers rise
and open, how
the pink lungs of their bodies
enter the fire of the world
and stand there shining
and willing...
—— Mary Oliver

Sequence 1: Breath and Action

The focus in this sequence is on stillness and the rhythm, quality, and duration of breath directly coordinated with physical action. The quality and duration of the breath determines the quality and duration of the action. You will begin at a slow and relaxed pace, pausing as frequently as you engage in physical action. This helps you not rush ahead or anticipate, and provides time to just notice what is happening in the present moment. The challenge in this exercise is to allow the breath to come in and out of the body naturally, without manipulating the duration of your inhale or exhale. Part I of this exercise can be a fast way to align attention, energy, and awareness. It is an excellent warm-up to most of the following exercises, to working with text, or performing on stage.

MOVING ON BREATH

1   Come into *Standing Alignment*. Close your eyes and focus on the rhythm of your breath. Do not change your breathing. Just notice your breath coming in and out of the body naturally as you stand in a relaxed state.

2   Notice the small pause — this moment of stillness — between your exhale and inhale.

3   Open your eyes and continue to focus on the rhythm of your breath. Again, do not interfere with your natural breathing — just notice it and breathe naturally.

4   Now begin to move easily for the duration of your exhale only. Pause as you inhale. These movements will be short, simple and relaxed, just as your exhale is short, simple and relaxed. You don't have to do much. Just turn your head, or raise your arm, curve your spine, or bend you knees. The rhythm of your natural breathing is determining the duration of your movement. Keep the breath and your movements relaxed.

5　Every time you exhale, move. Every time you inhale, be still. In the moments of stillness do not wait to move again, or anticipate your next gesture or movement. Give the same amount of attention and importance to the moments of stillness as to the moments of movement.

6　Relax into these full but brief moments of stillness. In stillness, tune in to how each of these unique shapes feel to you.

BREATHING RHYTHMS

You begin to address your expressive pallette and range by engaging in variations in the rhythm and quality of your breath. Instead of working directly on embodying emotions, by focusing on form — the breath and movement, in this case — emotions and internal states spontaneously arise. Through the next two exercises, you are encouraged to connect to your internal states as they arise as you move.

1　Now begin to change the rhythm of your breathing as you exhale. It can be a sudden burst of breath, slow and sustained, a series of percussive breaths, or any impulse that occurs to you.

2　Continue to move on your exhale only, matching the rhythm of your movement to the rhythm of your breath as exactly as possible. If your breath is a percussive burst, your movement is percussive. If your breath is slow and sustained, your movement is slow and sustained.

3　Remember to fully inhabit the moments of stillness as you inhale. You are not coming to neutral as you pause and inhale — you are simply ceasing to move your body.

BREATHING DYNAMICS

1   Now begin to play more with the dynamics of your breath, as well as the rhythm and duration of your breathing.

2   You can make your breath heavy and thick, light and airy, bouncy, sharp, smooth, rough, swirling, simple, complicated, tight, loose.

3   Match the quality and rhythm of your physical actions to the quality and rhythm of your breath. You do not have to match your movement directly to the duration of your exhale as in the previous exercises. Now you may move on your inhale too, but remember to find moments of stillness. This pause can now last for many breaths if you wish. Vary the duration of the physical actions and the pauses.

SOUND AND MOVE YOURSELF

Just as jazz musicians jam and improvise with their instruments, in this exercise you are going to be jamming with your body and voice. You are going to try to be as exacting as a musician in this exercise. You are going to directly line up your vocalization and your movements. The instant you sound, you move, and/or the instant you move you vocalize. When you are silent, you are still. It is as if the sound is animating the body, and the body is animating the sound. They happen at exactly the same time. You are also matching the dynamics of your movement and sound exactly — the rhythms, volume, tension level, and your inner state.

1   Begin by standing on your own, anywhere in the room.

2   You are going to begin by moving your hands and arms only.

3   Sound when you move, move when you sound, and pause in silence often. Your pause can extend beyond your inhale. You may pause for long and short periods of time. Play with a broad range of vocal dynamics and arm/hand movements, so voice and movement are the same speed, tempo, rhythm, energy, tension level, and dynamic.

4 Shift your vocal and physical dynamics often. Sometimes make your sound and movement soft, heavy and thick, smooth and long, short and percussive.

5 After a while, begin to engage more of your body. You can move through space. Remember that every time you move you are also making sound, and vica versa.

6 Keep changing the dynamics. Play with a large range of sounds and movements. Don't forget to interrupt your sound and movement with silence and stillness.

When facilitating this exercise, throw occasional suggestions out to the actors — fast, slow, smooth, rough, hard, soft, heavy, light, curvy, straight, percussive, low, high, oozy, sharp, sultry, tight, loose. Encourage students to continually experiment with changing dynamics.

This exercise is more difficult than it may seem as written here. To be aware of absolutely every movement — the exact moment one initiates a movement — and to match the exact dynamics with sound (and vice versa) is challenging. This practice helps build physical awareness, dynamic range, and congruence between our physical actions and our voice. It is an entrance to staying aware of the body while speaking.

Sequence 2: Sound and Action

SOUND AND ACTION CIRCLE

This is a simple exercise to do in a group. While standing in a circle, you will be passing sound and movement from person to person around the circle.

1 One person begins with a sound and movement, and that same sound and movement gets passed around the circle in a wave. You are not doing this to the person next to you, but sending your sound and movement into the center of the circle. There are no pauses between people as it gets passed around.

2 When that first sound and movement has been passed around the circle once and comes back to the originator, the next person in the circle creates a new, completely different sound and movement. It must contrast with the former sound and movement — energetically and physically — a wildly different sound, rhythm, duration, and dynamic.

3 For the person who originates the sound and movement, the practice is this: drop a breath into your center, and as you breathe out, allow a sound and movement to express itself. It is a small communication of an inner state or feeling that is expressing itself in this moment. These are short, primitive communications that may not make sense, or we may not know what they mean, but they are expressing something.

4 When it is your turn to originate a sound and movement, engage your whole body — spine, legs, arms, hips, and belly –and let your voice just come out. Don't plan what you are going to do. Just take a breath in and see what comes out. It is more fun to be surprised than to know what you are going to do!

As a sound and movement is passed around the circle, actors match the energy level of the originator of the sound and movement. It is an excellent way to discern who may be overly self-conscious, tends to lower the energy, has difficulty committing to the action, or slows the momentum down by pausing. When teaching, you can side-coach and encourage students to go further. It is also typical for younger actors to immediately drop out after they pass the sound and movement. Encourage them to sustain the moment of the feeling/sense of the sound and movement for a beat after they have passed it in the circle.

CONTRASTING SOUND AND ACTION

1   Repeat the previous exercise, *Movement and Sound Circle*.

2   Instead of passing one sound and one movement to the person next to you (similar to a one-syllable word), you are now going to offer two different, contrasting sounds and movements in quick succession (a two-syllable communication.)

ONE ACTION, ONE RESPONSE

1   Repeat *Sound and Action Circle* as a warm up.

2   Instead of passing a movement and sound around the circle, you are now going to slow it down and respond to one another's movements and sounds. This exercise can be done standing in a circle so all can experience each other's work, or it can be done in partners.

3   Partner A begins in the circle by offering a movement and sound to the person next to them, Partner B, in the circle. Partner A and B are not doing anything *to each other*, they are simply noticing each other and directing their actions towards each other in a small communication and exchange.

4   Your movement and sound is an expression of an inner state or feeling. You do not need to know what it is, or label it. But there is a mood, an inner atmosphere, or feeling state that inspires the action, and/or arises from the action.

5   Once Partner A has engaged in this movement and sound, they will pause in whatever shape and state they are in, breathe, and

notice Partner B. Remember that a *pause* is not a *freeze*. Partner A remains saturated in their state, open and breathing as Partner B responds with a contrasting action and sound.

6 Partner B in the circle is going to actively notice and experience Partner A as they breathe in. As Partner B exhales, they do a contrasting movement and sound in response to Partner A.

7 Partner B will then offer a new movement and sound to the person next to them (Partner C), and this process will continue around the circle a few times. Do not drop out between responding to your partner and offering a new, contrasting movement and sound to the next person in the circle.

Actors may initially be concerned about what it means *to respond* to another. We are always responding to something — an inner sense or feeling, a memory or association, other people, our environment — whether we are aware of it or not. If you are in an exchange with another person and genuinely taking them in, they affect you. Your actions will be a direct or indirect, an obvious or subtle expression of this.

EXTENDING THE ACTION

This is similar to *Sound and Action Circle*. Two people are simultaneously in two different movements and sounds, listening and responding to each other from inside of the experience. Together you orchestrate the separate rhythms of your individual actions and sounds in a simple communication and exchange.

1 While standing in a circle, one of you in the circle will begin by engaging in a movement and a sound.

2 This time, you are going to stay in the action by repeating your movement and sound. This is not a sound and movement that you are mechanically repeating. As you engage in this action, play with it a bit by experimenting with the rhythms, putting in long and short pauses, and noticing the details of the action you are in. It is mini-frame of an action.

3   The next person in the circle is going to respond to this action and sound. As the responder, you are going to notice what your partner is doing, and you will respond with a contrasting movement and sound. It will contrast in dynamics — your movement and sound will have a different dynamic quality, shape, rhythm, and tension level.

4   As you both engage in these two different frames of action, notice each other from inside of your frames. See if you can work off of each other, keeping the integrity of your own movement and sound. Pause inside your action for a moment, and notice your partner from this pause. Pause so you are not sounding over each other, but your voices and actions are interspersed and working together.

5   These are short interactions — less than a minute.

6   Now, the responder will do a new movement and sound, and the next person in the circle will respond.

7   Repeat this process around the circle.

Pausing in this exercise — suspending the sound and action — is important in order to listen and orchestrate your sound and movement with your partner. It takes practice to actively engage in an action and simultaneously listen and respond to another. The more you practice this exercise, the more tuned your listening becomes. You will become increasingly sensitive and responsive to the subtlest shifts in physical and vocal rhythms, and the energy and dynamics between you and your partner.

SOUND AND ACTION DUETS

This is similar to *Partner Interruptions* in Part Three: Sequence 2, but now you will add sound to the action.

1   This is an exchange of sound and actions. You will be working in partners. One of you engages in sound and movement until your partner interrupts you with a new sound and movement. Whenever you are interrupted, be still, breathe, and notice your partner. Do not come back to neutral. Just suspend your action and sound as your partner moves and sounds. Then interrupt them with a new sound and action.

2   You are both working in response to each other. You can move around the room, get close to each other, then far away.

3   Sometimes let your partner sound and move for awhile, sometimes interrupt them quickly. Keep changing the dynamics — the quality, rhythm, and tension level of your sound and action. Sometimes move slowly, sometimes quickly.

Sequence 3: Moving the Text

SOUND TO LANGUAGE

Words grab our attention. When we speak we usually focus primarily on the meaning of our words and our physical awareness tends to disappear. Content lies in what we say, in how we say it, and through our physical actions as we speak. This combination reveals our inner state, and effectively communicates an experience. In this exercise you begin to train your attention on *how* you are speaking — the rhythms, intonation, and sounds, and less on *what* you are saying — the meaning of your words.

This exercise can be done on your own, with a partner, or if facilitating this work, have the class stand in a circle and give each student a sound and action one at a time.

1   You will begin with a simple sound and action that you create on your own, or it can be provided to you by another.

2   Play with variations inside the frame until a word or phrase comes to you through association to the sound you are expressing.

3   When a word comes to you, begin to speak as you continue the action. As you speak, keep the integrity of the dynamics of the sound, and the sense or feeling of the sound quality, and stay in your action. Just speak a few sentences; then it is the next person's turn.

Here is an example:

With a simple movement I give the actor the sound "Whaaaa," with a specific dynamic and energy level. The actor begins to repeat that sound and action. Eventually an association will occur, and as soon as it does, they launch into language. It may sound something like this:

"Whaaa, whaaaa, whaaaaaaa, wha, whhhaaaaat, whaaat, whaaaaterr, whater, water! Whaater, there's whaaaater aaall around us. Wheee are on an island and the waaater is so blue!"

Another example: Begin with an action with the sound "Eeeeee":

The actor repeats and plays with the action and sound: "Eeee, eeeeee, eee, eeeeeeeve" until an association occurs: "Eeeevening, eeevening is heeeere. Oh, my! EEEEEEEE! Soooo dark. I can't seeeee anything! EEEEEEEK!"

Again, the speaking matches the sound and movement in intonation, rhythm, and feeling. It helps to pepper the words with the original sound from time to time. Play with the sound and action for as long as you need to for a word association to occur. It is apparent when one is over-thinking in this exercise, or attempting to think of something clever to say. Their voices will change immediately when they begin to speak words, and the feeling, sense, and movement will flatten. It really doesn't matter in this exercise what you say. The focus is on the vocal dynamics, the inner state the sound provokes in you, and keeping the body alive in the action as you speak.

LANGUAGE AND ACTION WITH A PARTNER

1   Partner A provides a simple Sound and Action.

2   Partner B joins A and does the same Sound and Action.

3   Once Partner B is doing the sound and action with the same dynamics and intention, Partner A stops to watch.

4   Partner B continues, and from the sound and action begins to speak. As in the previous exercise, *Sound to Language*, when you speak, keep the same intonation, dynamics, and sense of the original sound, and stay in the action.

5   The rhythm may change a bit. After you have done a short, physical narrative, stop. Switch roles.

Do this at least five or six times. This exercise helps develop a physically alive body and expressive voice. Once you become used to language that arises from the body, internal states, physical actions, vocal dynamics and words become more congruent and believable.

TEXT CIRCLE

This exercise is wonderful for working with heightened text, such as poetry or Shakespeare, but I have also applied it to contemporary dramatic texts with wonderful results. It can help sensitize you to the specific images, changing thoughts, and feelings in your text, while keeping the body active and alive. You can do this exercise before you have learned your text by heart, and it can be repeated after you have memorized your text.

To prepare for this exercise, look at your text and circle a few or all of the "big words and phrases" in the text — strong images, poetic words, or words that have layered meaning. This exercise can be done on your own, with a partner, or in a group. Put your printed text with circled words on the floor behind you.

Part I: One Word

Repeat the *Sound and Action Circle* (Sequence 1).

1   If working in a group, stand in a circle. If working with a partner, stand about six feet apart. Instead of sending a sound and action, you are now going to send a word from your text. You are going to sound and move that word — feel your way through the vowels and consonants. Move your whole body as you sound your way through the word and express the sense or feeling of that word. Experiment.

2   Begin by making eye contact with the person you are sending your word and movement to. Make sure your sound and movement makes its way to whomever you are sending it to — energetically, physically, and vocally. Don't forget to engage your whole body — legs, belly, chest, spine, and arms.

3   Similarly to *Sound and Action Circle*, the receiver will breath that word in, choose a new person in the circle, and respond with whatever word from their own text they have chosen.

4   Continue until everyone in the circle has sent and received a sound and movement word a few times.

5 Each time it is your turn to respond, try sounding and moving through your word with a different intention or feeling/sense. When you've done that a few times, try the next word from your text.

Part II: One Phrase

1 You will repeat the *One Word* exercise, but now you will send and receive a line of text, phrase, or sentence.

2 You are sounding and moving through each word of your line of text and sending it to another person in the circle. Each word has its own unique meaning and sound, and requires a different movement. Notice if you are over-engaging or putting extra tension in your arms, neck, and shoulders. See if you can connect to your center and stay grounded so you do not lean forward. Activate the lower half of your body — belly, hips, pelvis, legs, and spine — as you sound and move through your text.

Part III: Stand and Speak

1 You will take all that energy and intention of sounding and moving through your phrase and now bring it more into your core and spine. You will simply speak the phrase to someone in the circle instead of moving and sounding your way through it.

2 See if you can allow your body and voice to stay alive, and the words and images distinct and specific.

3 Try it again, this time speaking a few lines or sentences. Don't forget, you are responding to whatever text was sent to you by your partner or in a circle of people with your own text. Although your text will not make literal sense with whatever text was sent to you, you are working off of the energy that was sent to you. You are shifting from receiving text to offering your text to another person in the circle without dropping out in between. Imagine the text being sent to you is a wave of energy. You want to catch it at the top of the wave to begin speaking your text to keep the energy moving between you or in the circle of people you are working with.

I have noticed a significant difference in actors' text work after they do this sequence of exercises. It helps actors begin to build an active relationship to their text, and it makes learning their text by heart easier. It strengthens their personal and emotional connection to their text, and increases specificity and clarity. I also use this sequence when working with non-actors and beginning actors as a way to build a sense of ensemble, to get them speaking and listening on their feet together.

Moving on Breath, Eyes Follow the Action (Part Five: Sequence 1), *Sound and Movement Circle*, and *Text Circle* is a sequence I often employ at the beginning of rehearsals when I am directing. It can be done in less than 20 minutes. The sequence warms up the body and voice, gives actors time to tune into themselves and the text, and to come into relationship with each other. Whenever I take the time to do this before rehearsal begins, I notice a marked difference in actors' focus, energy, and work.

PART FIVE

The Body in Action

...Let us risk the wildest places,
Lest we go down in comfort, and despair.
— Mary Oliver

Sequence 1: The Eyes in Action

In this sequence you will focus on the eyes as an integral part of all of your actions. Our eyes are referred to as the gateway to the soul. Our eyes communicate our inner experience. From a relaxed to a heightened state, our eyes rapidly shift focus. Ask someone something as simple as what they had for breakfast, and their eyes usually move rapidly two or three times before they answer. Our eyes shift every time we have a fleeting thought, association, memory, feeling, or sensation. When there is excess tension, the eyes tend to freeze and lock onto one focal point. This is a common habit in audition and monologue work.

Actors need to be able to have multiple focal points on stage, and their focus and attention needs to be able to shift rapidly. This takes awareness and agility. Tension is constricting and inhibits this agility. Actors often lock eyes in scenes, and lock their eyes on one location as they deliver a monologue. In real life, we rarely do this.

In a minute of a scene on stage the actor may first be looking at their scene partner in an intimate exchange, then shift their focus up and outward as they grasp for a word or thought, then turn inward as they reflect, and back to their partner as they speak. Their eyes may dart from the floor to their partner's eyes as they listen, from side to side as they feel something, soften as they hear something they like, harden in defense, and on and on. We have a natural ability to do this and to hold multiple layers of awareness simultaneously if we are relatively relaxed and engaged.

When I consciously move my eyes as I move my body, I experience what feels like an instant hook-up with my internal states. My students have reported the same thing. After doing this exercise a few times, one of my students said it felt like he was given the keys to the kingdom — freer access to his feeling states and emotions. It is a simple technique that has been extremely effective in my students' work and has helped them strengthen the connection to their inner life.

EYES FOLLOW THE ACTION

1   You are going to be working with moving your eyes as well as your bodies. Allow your eyes to move in your eye sockets, instead of turning your whole head.

2   Similar to the exercise *Breath and Action* (Part Four: Sequence 2) you are working with the rhythm of your breath. You will move slowly and very simply for the duration of your exhale, and pause as you inhale. Do not change the natural rhythm of your breath. The movement and the pauses have the same weight and importance.

3   You will begin by just moving your arms. Your eyes will follow the direction of your movement. Do not look at your hands and arms, but follow the direction of your movement with your eyes — if you move your arms to the side, your eyes move in that direction. Keep your head still, and just move your eyeballs.

4   Besides looking up, down, to the sides, and on the diagonals, you can also gaze far away, in a medium range, turn your gaze inward, and behind you.

5   After you have experimented with this for a while begin to engage other parts of your body. Pause on your inhale, and move for the duration of your exhale.

EYES CONTRAST THE ACTION

1   You are going to start at the beginning again, just moving our arms. This time, instead of following the action with your eyes, you are going to contrast it. For instance, if you move your arms down, your eyeballs will look upward. If you move your arms forward, you will put your gaze in the back of your head.

2   This may feel awkward, as our gaze tends to follow the action naturally. Remember to keep your head still and just move the eyes. Do not push or muscle your eye movements. Keep your eyes relaxed.

3 When you feel acclimated, begin to move different body parts or in any way you wish. Remember to pause as you inhale.

4 Now, sometimes follow the direction of your movements with your eyes and sometimes contrast.

If working in a group, divide the class in half to watch. The amount of images, attitudes, and feelings that are expressed in this exercise can be surprising. Students easily see the power of the eyes, and the myriad nuanced inner states they express.

LINING IT UP

1 You are going to play with the rhythm and quality of your breath and your movement, but now you are going to continue to keep your eyes active. Sometimes you will move quickly, sometimes very slowly, sometimes in fast stops and starts, sometimes in little micro movements. You can make your movements and the quality of your breath heavy, soft, thick, light, complicated, or simple. Move any way you wish and experiment with different rhythms and dynamics.

2 You are matching the quality of your eyes to the quality of your breath and movement. You can make your eyes sharp, diffuse, soft, hard, distant, close, delicate, strong, or any way you wish.

3 Don't worry about whether you are following or contrasting the direction of your movement with your eyes. Just be aware of your eyes.

4 Keep changing the dynamics, and don't forget to pause — to find these full moments of stillness.

5 Notice how you are feeling, and what images arise as you move. See if these inform what you are doing and how you are doing it.

Keeping the eyes engaged is reinforced in all of the subsequent exercises. After you have done these exercises a few times, it only requires a quick reminder to engage the eyes. When you do engage your eyes, you may notice that you feel more committed to your actions and more connected to your internal states and feelings. Your communicative impact increases noticeably when you engage your eyes.

STEPPING STATES

Because of the tension that can accompany performing, actors often plant themselves in one place and stand with arms at their sides. In real life, our internal states, energy, and tension level constantly shift, and our bodies animate naturally in response. This can be layered, nuanced, and subtle. It may be a small increase or decrease of tension in the spine or chest, a slight movement of the shoulders and head or change in eye focus. This exercise begins to increase awareness of these ever changing internal states, and gets the physical systems jump-started and re-accustomed to energy moving through it, so the body animates naturally in concert with the fluidity of our ever-changing internal states.

Remember the *Expand and Fold* exercise (Part I: Sequence 5) and the sense of incrementally filling yourself up with energy, draining energy out from the core of the body, and allowing that action to initiate movement. In this exercise you will bring extra awareness to the eyes and face. You are simultaneously filling up the core of the body, and initiating movement in the eyes and face.

If working in a group, line up side-by-side at the back of the studio. Slowly step forward until you reach the front of the room. After doing the exercise once, divide the group in half to watch each other.

1   In this exercise you are very slowly filling yourself up with energy and very slowly draining energy out of the body. You are simultaneously initiating your movement with the eyes and with your facial muscles. Move slowly.

2   You are going to walk forward slowly and at an even pace. Every time your foot hits the ground, you are going to pause for just a moment. It is like a quick, still picture, in which you stop your

action and notice where you are on the continuum of filling up and draining out.

3 Engage your lips, mouth, jaw, forehead, cheeks, and nose. Move your eyes.

4 Every time your foot hits the ground, your eyes will be focused in a new direction, the tension level in your body and facial expression will change.

5 Try to keep your walking even and slow. Don't forget to pause a moment when you have stepped forward and your foot is on the floor.

Sequence 2: Framing the Action

Working in frames is a skill and technique that is central to the practice of Action Theater. You began to work in mini-frames in *Sound and Action* (Part Four: Sequence 3). In this sequence you do a version of *Shifting Frames* in preparation for working with text. The focus when working in frames is on the form, or the details of the physical action. Emotions, characters, and stories may arise, but the practice is to focus on the physical details of the action. Frames are a way to bracket a moment in time — to notice, explore, and express the details of that moment. They are not like a picture frame, but more like a microscope focused on something living. Every inner state has a specific energetic quality, dynamic, tension level, rhythm, and form. The physical elements and accompanying inner state in a frame do not change, but the subtle rhythms and movements within a frame are ever-changing.

In this work we generally refer to inner states, rather than emotions. An inner state is a feeling, sense, or inner atmosphere. It is slightly broader and more inclusive than working exclusively with emotions. In our daily lives we sense and feel something, and then an emotion may arise, with associations, thoughts, and memories, which inform our actions. All of these levels of experience are usually going on at the same time. As I discussed in Part Two: The Intuitive Body, in acting exercises when an emotion arises, there is a tendency to get tense, physically constrict, and to get overly attached to the emotion. Young actors often confuse emoting with acting, or attempt to play emotions rather than actions. When this happens, their acting work suffers and their physical awareness drops away.

Conceptualizing and working in frames clarifies action and the intention behind an action. It is a way to stay awake and responsive to the physical details, whether moving, standing still, and/or speaking. The action informs the inner state and the inner state informs the action when working within a frame. You do not begin with an idea, emotion, situation or character. You always begin with an action — a movement, shape, gesture — large or small, moving or not. You then focus on the details, dynamics, rhythm and form of that action, and open your awareness to the inner state this action awakens and inspires. This way of working encourages you to avoid working imitatively, helps you address habitual associations and responses, and allows you to make new discoveries.

If you stop and notice what you are doing at this moment while reading this — the position of your body, the rhythm of your breath, tension level in the body, and even the smallest movement in your eyes, toes, mouth, or hands, and then deepen into the details of all of this — perhaps exaggerate it a little — this is a frame. You are experiencing and communicating a particular inner atmosphere, state, or feeling. Right now, shift your body into a new position. Change the tension level in your body. Change where your eyes are focused and the rhythm of your breath. You are now in a new frame that communicates a different state from the frame you were just in. We are always in frames of action that communicate an inner state, mood, feeling or emotion.

In life, we shift frames often. Sometimes it is subtle, sometimes it is not. If I am slowly strolling down a country path, arms gently swinging, calmly taking in the air and sights around me, I am in a specific frame of action. My actions and the energy, rhythm, and dynamics of my actions express a particular mood, atmosphere, or feeling. If I suddenly hear a growl in the woods as I am walking, I might suddenly stop, hold very still, my spine might straighten upward as my eyes dart around. I have just *shifted* into a new *frame* — a new shape, dynamic, and rhythm — a completely new inner state.

Shifting Frames encourages clarity, specificity, and physical responsiveness. Applied directly to working with text, actors gain skills in tracking, responding, and communicating the beats in a text — the shifting moods, thoughts, and images, with more specificity, clarity, and agility. It encourages a physically awake body while speaking, and an ability to make both subtle and bold physical choices.

SHIFTING FRAMES

Part I

You can do this exercise on your own, with a partner, or in a group. If facilitating this exercise, inform the group that you will be giving them a series of fast directions: within those directions they will be asked to go into a frame of *Sound and Action* (Part Four: Sequence 3). In other words, they will notice whatever shape and state they are in, and that will be their frame, or starting place, to explore that action and inner state with sound and movement. A frame is an action or series of movements that express an inner state, mood, or atmosphere. You are not mechanically repeating a sound and movement, but exploring the details within a specific frame of action and state of mind.

1 Change your location in the room.

2 Change your facing in the room.

3 Change your shape. Just throw your body into a shape.

4 Change your shape again.

5 Keep that shape, but change where your eyes are focused.

6 Take this into a *Sound and Action Frame.*

7 Explore this frame for a minute or two. Keep the rhythm within your action varied and pause within your frame from time to time. In the pause, you do not drop out. You are still saturated in whatever inner state you are in, your eyes are active and you are breathing. You have simply suspended the physical action for a moment.

8 Stop. Change your location in the room again.

9 Change your shape.

10 Keep this shape, but change the tension level inside of you.

11 Change the position of your arms and hands.

12 Change your eye focus.

13 Take this into a frame of movement only — no sound.

Repeat these directions, or a combination of similar directions many times, alternating *Sound and Action Frames*, or *Movement Only Frames* of action. When facilitating this exercise I usually go around the room and do individual side-coaching, encouraging actors to go further, more deeply into the details of what they are doing, and to breathe.

Part II

1   When working with a partner, one of you will call "Shift." or if facilitating this work, you will call "Shift" to the group. Each time you hear "shift, you will change your *frame* — your shape, action, tension level, rhythm, and dynamic quality.

2   Each time you shift, you will be in a completely new frame that contrasts the frame you were just in. As you work within a frame, deepen into the details of what is already happening internally and in your actions. Notice what you are doing, feeling, sensing; how you are in the space, the rhythm, and quality of your action.

3   Remain in and explore the details of each frame until you hear "Shift."

SHIFTING FRAMES:
MOVEMENT, SOUND, AND LANGUAGE

1   Repeat *Shifting Frames*. At a certain point when you are in a *Movement Only Frame* or *Movement and Sound Frame*, you are going to add language to your frame. It is surprising how easily improvised language can come to you when you are engaged in a frame.

2   When teaching this work you will call out "Shift," and alternate instructing actors to enter frames that are *Movement Only*, *Sound and Movement*, and *Movement and Language*.

3   After you have guided actors through this exercise for about 10 minutes, they can shift on their own (without you calling "Shift"). Instruct them to alternate *Movement Only*, *Sound and Movement*, and *Movement and Language Frames* as they wish.

There are many ways to practice *Shifting Frames*. In a class you can practice in partners, taking turns watching each other: one is the "director" who calls "Shift." You can partner students to go into each other's frames: one is the provider and one is the follower. The provider enters a frame of any combination of movement, sound and/or language, and their partner enters that frame with them. This is called *Simultaneous Shifting* — two people doing the same thing at the same time. You are not mirroring each other, but playing together within the same frame, working with and off of each other.

Shifting through a monologue can be a useful preparatory technique that helps clarify the beats in a dramatic text. This can feel a little mechanical, but it helps keep energy and breath moving through the body while speaking. Once you Shift through your text with bold choices, you can do it a second time more subtly, such as simply shifting your eye focus, the tension level in your spine or facing in the room.

Sequence 3:
Introduction to Character Dynamics

When working on monologues, scenes, or a play, I tend to move between text work and physical, nonverbal work. Going back and forth between the spoken word and the speaking body helps actors strengthen the connection between their inner world, physical life, expressive actions, and the spoken word.

BODY CENTERS

In this sequence you will collapse, suspend, and lead from specific centers of the body. As you play with your physical alignment, you will allow the rest of your body to do whatever it wants to do, and notice any associations and feelings that arise.

You will walk around the room, stand still, turn, gesture, and sit in a chair as you wish. Again, allow yourself to freely associate whatever inner states arise from these adjustments in your alignment: How old do you feel? What is your attitude towards the others in the room and the world? How are you using space — boldly, timidly, staying at the side of the room, walking in curves or straight lines? What is your rhythm: are you moving slowly, quickly, in a sustained or percussive way?

If facilitating this work, add these prompts while actors explore. Encourage them to exaggerate what they are doing at times (going into caricature) and then to make very subtle choices, and everything in between. You may wish to encourage your students to play with gestures (fixing their clothes, or social gestures such as waving "hello," etc.).

Explore each instruction for at least 5 minutes. I have added in parentheses possible associations one might have when engaged in this exercise. Although these kinds of prompts can be useful, if facilitating this work I suggest you keep these kinds of prompts as open and varied as possible so actors can have their own personal associations.

A good warm-up into this exercise is *Isolations* (Part One: Sequence 1).

1 Focus on your head. Raise your chin just a little, and begin to walk around the room. Notice what this feels like. Allow the rest of your body to respond to whatever associations or feelings arise. (Are you looking down your nose at the world? Are you feeling eager? Straining upwards?)

2 Stop. Now push your chin down slightly. See what this feels like as you walk, stand, sit, gesture. (Are you looking through your brow at the world? Are you a little shy and withdrawn?)

3 Now push your whole face forward. See what the rest of your body does in response to this. (Are you straining forward into the world? Eager? Looking for connection?)

4 Stop and stand still. Now focus on your heart center — the center of your chest. Push this area of the body straight down. Explore. (Do you feel tired? Old? Withdrawn or shy? Sad? Low energy?)

5 Now push the center of your chest up, as if you were holding yourself up from your heart center. (Do you feel important? Guarded? Male or female? Tense? Old? Young?)

6 Push your heart center forward into the world and lead from this center. (Do you feel as if you are straining into the world? Do you want something? Do you feel young or old? Male or female?)

7 Press your pelvis forward and lead from this area of the body. Notice what the rest of your body wants to do in response to this adjustment.

8 Now tuck your tailbone under, subtly rounding your lower back (like a dog with his tail between his legs).

The subtlest shifts in physical alignment can powerfully express the inner life, attitude, and psychological make-up of a character. It can also be an introduction to further exploration of historic period manners and deportment — to help actors' awareness of their contemporary and perhaps more casual style and habits.

I have also applied this exercise to help sensitize actors to their habits of alignment and to help tune them into the psychophysical aspects of alignment. As discussed in Part One, your history and psychological make-up affects your alignment, and your alignment can affect your energy, how you perceive and are perceived by others. If facilitating this work, you may wish to introduce it after completing Part One: Sequence 1.

DIRECT/INDIRECT

Part I

In this part of the exercise you can only do one thing at a time, and your action must be very clear. Begin with *Standing Alignment* (Part One: Sequence 1).

1 Stand anywhere in the room. Ground and center yourself, and breathe. Turn just your head to focus on a specific place across the room.

2 Keep you eyes on your focal point and turn your whole body to face that direction.

3 Ground and center yourself again.

4 Walk to whatever you are focused on in a direct line crossing the room. Keep your pace fairly slow and sustained, and keep your eyes on your focal point. Feel the floor underneath you and be aware of the ceiling above you as you cross the room.

5 Come to a complete stop when you arrive at the place you were focused on and point to it or touch it if it is within reach.

6 Come back into Standing Alignment, arms at your side.

7 Turn your head to focus on a new place across the room. Repeat.

After you have gone through 1–7 a few times, add:

8 As you are walking to whatever focal point you have, stop and do a simple but large gesture, such as bringing your arms to your chest and extending both arms outward. Be aware of your eye focus as you gesture, and stay in a relatively slow and sustained rhythm as you gesture. Complete your gesture by bringing both arms back down to your sides. Then continue to walk to your focal point.

Beware of rushing ahead and doing more than one action at a time, like turning your head and body at the same time, or turning the body and walking immediately, without taking the time to ground and center yourself. This exercise is one action at a time!

Part II

1 You are going to repeat this exercise, but now you will blur the line between your actions. You might get distracted halfway across the room and need to fix your hair or clothes, fidget, forget what you are supposed to be doing, or get distracted by another person and follow them across the room to their focal point.

2 Instead of being in a slow or sustained rhythm, your rhythm might be erratic, with sudden stops and starts. Your eye focus might change rapidly. As in Part One, after you have done the sequence a few times, try stopping as you cross the room to gesture. Play with small gestures that do not extend far from the body.

PERSONAL SPACE

There is a tendency, especially with young actors, to crowd each other in scene work and onstage. Stage space should remain open to include the audience, and so the space does not collapse between characters onstage. Each individual has their own sense of personal space, informed by their age, psychological make-up, history, culture, and era in which they were born. The following exercise can begin to deepen your awareness of personal space.

1   Stand across a room facing a partner, with lots of space between you. Come into *Standing Alignment* (Part One: Sequence 1) and allow your breath to drop into your center.

2   Remember the easy eye focus in the *Walking and Stillness* exercise (Part Three: Sequence 1) where you allow energy out of the eyes with a sense of receiving, rather than pushing or grabbing with your eyes. Allow your eyes to rest on your partner's eyes for the duration of this exercise.

3   Partner A will stand still (the Receiver). Partner B will walk very slowly towards Partner A (the Approacher).

4   Try to remain relaxed, receptive, and centered as you are approaching or being approached. Stay focused on each other, breathe, and notice when you get distracted or want to fidget.

5   At any point the Approacher can stop to ground and center themselves, or the Receiver can put their hand up to communicate to the Approacher to stop for a moment.

6   As you get closer to each other, you both should notice a subtle but palpable shift in the energy between you. This is usually when you are on the edge or have just stepped into each other's personal space.

7   When the Approacher senses this moment, stop, take a few steps backwards, and then continue forward again. Keep approaching your partner until you are about a foot apart.

8   Switch roles.

Leave time after you have both been the Receiver and the Approacher to talk to your partner about their experience of the exercise.

Once you have done this exercise a few times, you can apply it to scene work. Try going through your scene with an awareness of personal space. Experiment with respecting and breaking each other's personal space: you can try standing behind your scene partner, very close or across the room, walking away, turning your back to each other, facing the diagonal. This type of experimentation with personal space can inform your interpersonal dynamics and have a profound dramatic impact.

The following sequence of exercises is useful for experimenting with personal space. It can also be used as an introduction to exploring status relationships in scenes and plays. Personal space is a major status indicator. An obvious example is that a servant would never get too close to a queen. Touching another person, like putting a hand on someone's shoulder while speaking, can indicate familiarity and affection, or it can be subtly condescending and immediately lower the social status of the person being touched. How two people are in relationship to each other spatially in private may change in a public setting or formal social occasions.

Sequence 4: Clear Action

BEGIN/END

The focus of this exercise is to make specific, clear choices. The movement pallette is paired down to ordinary, everyday, human movement. You respond to your partner from a sense, feeling, instinct, or impulse, as opposed to a thought or idea.

In *Begin/End* you work with subtle, simple gestures and actions. The smallest action — from a slight turn of the head, a movement of the eyes, a shift in weight, changing the angle and distance of the body in relationship to another, or the smallest adjustment in your physical alignment — has profound communicative power.

1   Stand facing a partner. You are going to be working in response to your partner with a very simple, ordinary movement palette. You will not engage in physical contact with your partner.

2   Each time you respond, you will just do one, very simple and clear action.

3   Before you begin any action, you will say "begin" out loud. When you have completed your one action you will say "end." When you have ended your action, stay in whatever position you are in, breathe, and take in your partner, who will respond.

4   Keep your movement very simple. Just one simple action at a time — like turning your head, sinking into one hip, taking one step, reaching, crossing your arms, turning to face a new direction — always bookended by saying "begin" and "end." You do not have to make anything happen, or do anything clever or significant. All you have to do is notice your genuine responses to your partner's simple actions — just notice, experience, and respond with a simple choice.

5   What does it feel like to reach your hand out to your partner and have them turn their back to you, or reach towards you? What does it feel like to lock eyes, or avert your eyes to avoid your partner's gaze? Step in closer or move farther away? Look down or up at your partner? Again, keep your actions simple and just notice what is happening between you. Do not rush.

6 If you feel disengaged, try upping the ante a bit by making a bolder choice or direct offer to your partner. Accepting your partner's offer does not mean that you are always agreeable. See what it feels like to turn your back on your partner, walk away, or move in very close.

7 Allow the dynamics between you to constantly shift. Don't get stuck in one dynamic, scenario, idea, or story.

This exercise encourages trust in the expressive power of simple choices, and the degree to which we communicate through body language. This is a good exercise to use as a warm-up into scene work. For some actors it is challenging to not *make something happen* in this exercise. When facilitating this work I notice actors tend to initially engage in a lot of facial expressions, social gestures (such as waving "hi" or shaking their head "no"), or pantomime. In this exercise you just need to notice what is already happening inside of you and between you and your partner(s), instead of forcing any content or enacting any scenarios. My students are often surprised by the immediacy of their responses, and the variety of genuine emotions these simple and nonverbal interactions provoke.

BEGIN/END DYNAMICS

You can repeat this exercise two or three times, pairing up with different partners. You can also do the exercise with three people. There is a wonderful tension in working in odd numbers like trios. Similar to many of these exercises, you focus on form — how you are engaging in an action — and then notice the resulting inner atmosphere, mood, feeling, or emotional response this inspires in you.

1 Repeat the *Begin/End* exercise. This time pay extra attention to the rhythm of your actions. Sometimes go slowly. Sometimes hesitate inside of your actions, or make your actions direct, or fast and sharp. Put small pauses in your actions, or pause between when you say "begin" and when you move. See how this changes what you are doing and experiencing, or inspires a different response from your partner. Still stay tuned into each other. Everything you do is in direct response to your partner.

2 Repeat the exercise again. This time be aware of the different centers of your body — head, heart, solar plexus, and pelvis. Work with extra awareness of these different areas of the body. What does it feel like to collapse your heart center? To turn your pelvis away from your partner? To crane your head towards them as you pull your heart center back? To initiate an action with your head?

3 Repeat the exercise again, and pay extra attention to your spatial relationship. What does it feel like slowly approach your partner? To quickly move away? To approach them from behind? To come right up to their face? To walk away?

I notice that after actors experiment in this exercise a number of times, their actions and responses become more specific, nuanced, and subtle. This exercise illuminates social behavior and a variety of interpersonal dynamics. After actors have explored *Begin/End*, I often divide the group to watch. This is a good entrance to observing and discussing body language, gesture, and status indicators.

My students tend to have a variety of strong responses to the dynamics they see occurring between actors in this exercise. When facilitating this work, the more you can help your students break down why they are having these responses — what the actors they are observing are *specifically doing* that inspires their responses — the more your students can begin to understand body language and its power to communicate. Our words are a small percentage of our communication. We unconsciously receive more information from a person's manner, energy, appearance, and body language than from what they are saying. Actors need to familiarize themselves with the rich world of gesture and body language. These exercises provide an introduction to continued study in this area.

BEGIN/END IN CHAIRS

I make a distinction in my classes between performing in front of the class and volunteering to experiment in front of the class. In this exercise only two actors experiment at a time as the rest of the class observes.

1   You do this exercise with a partner, sitting in chairs angled obliquely towards each other. You are still working within the guidelines of the previous exercises, but you no longer say "begin" and "end" out loud. You do, however, keep your responses to a single, clear action and will work in direct response to your partner's actions.

2   You will continue to work in a palette of ordinary actions, such as turning your body towards and away from your partner, leaning into your partner's personal space, crossing a leg, turning your head, and various opened and closed physical positions.

3   Take your time to notice and experience your partner's action before you respond.

Again, this exercise offers a framework to investigate, explore, and discuss body language. When directing or working on scenes, this exercise can be used to explore the interpersonal dynamics between characters. Actors do the exercise and make their choices based on what they understand about their characters' status, objectives, psychology, and interpersonal dynamics with their scene partner. It can also be a useful exercise for actors to explore a movement pallette appropriate to the social manners and styles of specific cultures and historic time periods.

SILENT SCENES

Building on *Begin/End in Chairs*, the physical actions become more varied in *Silent Scenes*. You will work specifically with a character within the framework of a scene from a play.

Although you are working within the framework of a specific character and scene, you are not enacting the literal actions of your scene. You are improvising with your scene partner, exploring your character and interpersonal dynamics with your scene partner.

1   You will be given a set of actions to begin, that either you or your scene partner can do at anytime. You then add your own actions that arise in response to your scene partner's actions. Allow yourself to indulge whatever impulses arise.

2   The initial set of actions can be altered depending on the scene. The following is an example: An entrance, an approach, a reach towards your scene partner (with your hand, heart, or face), sitting down, circling each other, crossing the room, looking out a window, dealing with a prop (pouring a drink, putting on a shawl, putting on lipstick, etc.).

This improvisation can help deepen what you have discovered through more traditional rehearsal methods, and what you understand through your research and first impressions of a character, scene or play. Freed from language, and working with impulse and instinct, you can go deeper and often discover a variety of subtle dynamics.

A FEW WORDS ON TEACHING

Actor's bodies are their instruments. In teaching movement, we are also guiding students in a process of self-discovery. Students of acting come up against physical, emotional, and mental habits that are potentially limiting. Actors tend to be overly self-critical and expert on their limitations. Resistance, judgment, and frustration in class are not uncommon. When teaching this work, providing ways to examine and move past limiting habits, and encouraging curiosity can ease this tendency. A healthy amount of joy and humor in the classroom also helps. Continually guiding actors' attention on action is, of course, more helpful than pointing out what they are not doing. Encouragement, respect, and individual guidance are key.

Acting students learn from the way in which instructors embody the principles they teach. Students take their cues from the tone in which an instructor sets up an exercise. The atmosphere can be light, playful, energetic, serious, or meditative. How an exercise is introduced and framed, where instructors guide students' attention through verbal prompts or hands-on work, and the words and images the instructor employs are essential to actors' experience and growth. For this reason, I have been as specific as possible in each sequence of exercises. I cannot overemphasize the importance of employing images when teaching this work, and encouraging actors to utilize their mind's eye. Images are more than mental pictures, and the mind's eye is multisensory. We use both to direct attention and activate this all-important connection between the senses, feelings, imagination, and action.

Just as precision in the teacher's language is important, so is the actors' ability to verbally articulate their observations, impressions, and experiences of the work. It is useful to talk briefly after the exercises, or at the end of class. This helps actors synthesize and integrate the work. In my classes, we practice speaking from the personal — employing "I" instead of the common "you." We make a distinction between "I sensed," "I imagined," "I felt," "I thought," and collectively unpack the meaning behind general, nondescriptive words that are commonly employed such as "interesting" or "weird." This helps students begin to speak *from* their experience instead of *about* it, which is a useful practice for all actors.

Establishing an expansive, disciplined, and safe environment in which to work is essential to support students' ability to explore, take risks, and venture collectively into the unknown. A healthy studio environment is an active undertaking based on understanding and respect for the work and each other. My expectation as a teacher of movement and improvisation for actors is that I am in a room of artists who take themselves seriously, and who are equally passionate about their work and the creative process. I remind my students that they are entering and participating in a long and rich tradition.

A transition between the outside world and the studio is helpful. The ritual of changing into workout clothing, turning cell phones off, clearing the space, and sweeping the floors are all useful transitional activities for students. The sense is of leaving a bit of the ordinary world out there to make room for the extraordinary. I ask students to arrive early to prepare for class. Once they enter the studio, I request that they speak quietly or not at all, and take the time to stretch, breathe, and check-in with themselves. This creates an atmosphere of ease and focus in the room before we gather to begin class. From the instant students enter the studio for the duration of the working session, they are practicing and exercising their "muscle" of awareness. The message is: in here, anything can happen. And it does!

SUGGESTED READING

Contact Improvisation:

Contact Quarterly: Dance & Improvisation Journal
https://contactquarterly.com

Action Theater:

Zaporah, Ruth. *Improvisation on the Edge*. Berkeley: North Atlantic Books, 2014.

Zaporah, Ruth. *Action Theater: The Language of Presence*. Berkeley: North Atlantic Books, 1995.

Action Theater/Zap Performance Projects:
http://www.actiontheater.com

Body-Mind Centering:

Cohen, Bonnie Bainbridge. *Sensing, Feeling, and Action: The Experiential Anatomy of Body-Mind Centering*. Northampton: Contact Editions, 1997.
http://www.bodymindcentering.com

Authentic Movement:

Adler, Janet. *Offering from the Conscious Body: The Discipline of Authentic Movement*. Rochester: Inner Traditions, 2002.

Alexander Technique:

Gelb, Michael. *Body Learning*. New York: Holt Publishers, 1994.

Movement For Actors:

Potter, Nicole, Ed. *Movement for Actors*. New York: Allworth Press, 2002

Wangh, Stephen. *An Acrobat of the Heart*. New York: Vintage Books, 2000.

Marshall, Lorna, and Oida, Yoshi. *The Body Speaks*. New York: Palgrave MacMillan, 2002.

Polatin, Betsy. *The Actor's Secret*. Berkeley: North Atlantic Books, 2013.

Tea With Trish: The Movement Work of Trish Arnold (DVD)
http://www.teawithtrish.com

Merry Conway: http://www.merryconway.com

CPSIA information can be obtained
at www.ICGtesting.com
Printed in the USA
BVHW05s2358100818
523711BV00003B/25/P